THE
Fast Track
ONE-DAY
Detox Diet

Boost Metabolism,
Get Rid of Fattening Toxins,
Safely Lose up to 8 Pounds Overnight
and Keep Them Off for Good

Ann Louise Gittleman, Ph.D., C.N.S.

MORGAN ROAD BOOKS
New York

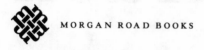

MORGAN ROAD BOOKS

Published by Morgan Road Books, an imprint of The Doubleday Broadway Publishing Group, a division of Random House, Inc.

Disclaimer: This book is not intended to take the place of medical advice from a trained medical professional. Readers are advised to consult a physician or other qualified health professional regarding treatment of their medical problems. Neither the publisher nor the author takes any responsibility for any possible consequences from any treatment, action, or application of medicine, herb, or preparation to any person reading or following the information in this book.

PRINTED IN THE UNITED STATES OF AMERICA

Morgan Road Books and the M colophon are trademarks of Random House, Inc.

Visit our Web site at www.morganroadbooks.com

First edition published 2005

Book design by Lee Fukui

Library of Congress Cataloging-in-Publication Data
Gittleman, Ann Louise.
    The fast track one-day detox diet : boost metabolism, get rid of fattening toxins, safely lose up to 8 pounds over night and keep them off for good / Ann Louise Gittleman.
        p. cm.
    1. Detoxification (Health) 2. Weight loss. I. Title.
RA784.5.G58 2005
613.2'5—dc22

                                                                                            2004065606

ISBN 0-7679-2045-7

10   9   8   7   6

For Daniel Ryan Gittleman,
a most extraordinary young boy who has
blessed the Gittleman family

Acknowledgments

Grateful acknowledgment goes to *Woman's World* magazine, which planted the seed for this book in the first place. My most grateful thanks also to Wendy Meyerson, owner extraordinaire of Natur-Tyme in East Syracuse, New York, and to Laurel Sterling Prisco, R.D., for organizing the hundred dieters who were the original focus group for this project. Wendy, my offer still holds. I would hire you in a New York minute. Wendy's late father, Stan Meyerson, was a dear friend of mine, and I know how proud he would be of his daughter's business and marketing acumen.

I must also thank Rachel Kranz, my miracle muse, for her 24/7 devotion to this book, which was written in record time. Rachel, there are no words to express how much I appreciate your commitment, creativity, and warmth. You were always upbeat—whether we spoke at dawn or dusk or in the wee hours of the morning. What a pleasure!

Major kudos to my literary agent, Coleen O'Shea, who was also my editor for my first book in 1988. I am truly very happy that we are together again and I am definitely looking forward to many more projects together. You have been a guiding light and a voice of reason in so many ways. It's nice to be back in your capable hands, and thanks for all the tender loving care you have extended to me and my projects.

Thank you to the entire Morgan Road imprint. From the very beginning, Doubleday Broadway president and publisher Stephen Rubin, associate publisher and executive director of marketing Jackie Everly-Warren, and senior editor Phyllis Grann got on board with enthusiasm and passion. Amy Hertz, my publisher, caught the vision of this book, as have Catherine Pollock, the director of marketing, Suzanne Herz, associate publisher and executive director of publicity, Laura Pillar, senior publicist, and Marc Haeringer, associate editor. You have all collectively reignited my own excitement about health and the possibilities for transformation that this book embodies.

The recipes in this book were a labor of love. My thanks are extended to Catherine Ziegler and recipe mavens and cooks Linda Shapiro and Charli Sorenson. Linda Alexander, a devoted friend and cook, assisted me with the delicious task of taste-testing.

On the home front, I must sincerely thank my personal trainer, Rex Lettau, who fit me in and let me vent my creative frustrations during our one-on-one weight-training sessions. And of course Stuart Gittleman, my business and operations manager, who never let an interview or important e-mail slip by throughout the writing of this book. Stuart is my brother and we enjoy a very rare and unique business relationship and have for nearly ten years. Has it been that long, Stu?

I would like to take this opportunity to personally thank and acknowledge the people in the natural foods industry who have been longtime supporters of my work. Much love and thanks to Debra Stark in Concord, Massachusetts; Al Forman in Coral Springs, Florida; David and Sandy Gerhardt in Marietta, Georgia; Mary Legg in Stratford, Connecticut; Barbara Hoffmann in Wichita, Kansas; Joe Hamilton in Coeur d'Alene, Idaho; Marlene Beadle in Tacoma, Washington; Patti Milligan in Scottsdale, Arizona; Mary Mulry of Wild Oats; Nancy Huey of Henry's Market Place; Gene Greenfield of Whole Foods; and anyone else I may have inadvertently missed. I am also so grateful to Debbie Nelson-Judd, R.N., for her professional support and insights. Thank you, Deb, for your extraordinary work ethic and lovely spirit.

Finally, thanks to James, my personal hero, for his patience, love, and wisdom. You have created a healing home of health, wholeness, and love for us that enables me to recharge on a daily basis. Forever is as far as I'll go . . .

Contents

THE

Fast Track
ONE-DAY
Detox Diet

Get on the Fast Track!

*Each progressive spirit is opposed by a thousand
mediocre minds appointed to guard the past.*
—Maurice Maeterlinck

What if you could lose 3 to 8 pounds in a single day?

What if that nearly instant weight loss made you feel lighter, freer, cleaner, and more energized?

What if that one day of weight loss could help jump-start a long-term weight-loss plan? What if that single day began a healing, cleansing, revitalizing process, raising your awareness of the poisons that pollute our environment and purging your body of the toxins that set you up for weight gain, fatigue, and a host of deadly, debilitating diseases?

Well, that single day is here. It's called the Fast Track One-Day Detox Diet. It's safe. It feels terrific. And it works.

A One-Day Miracle Diet: Too Good to Be True?

Who doesn't like quick fixes and magic bullets? They're the reason that weight-loss products promising instant results have become a multibillion-dollar industry that's growing every year. The fact that most of these trendy diets don't work, don't last, and often put us at risk for serious health problems seems less important to many desperate dieters than the glittering promises these plans make.

As a nutritional maverick, I have always bucked the system Yet for more than twenty years, even I believed that there's no such thing as a magic bullet—although my internationally best-selling *Fat Flush Plan* has certainly come close! Throughout my hands-on experience with thousands of patients and clients in the public health arena (including a stint as the chief nutritionist for the pediatric clinic at New York City's Bellevue Hospital) and in the private sector (several years as the director of nutrition at the Pritikin Longevity Center in Santa Monica, California), I've always advocated long-term lifestyle changes, avoiding the one-shot answers that seem so popular in the weight-loss world. Although many diet gurus preached the gospel of exercising more and eating less, of cutting out fats, or—more recently—of eliminating carbs, I've always understood that our bodies and metabolisms are too complex for such simple solutions.

When I introduced my two-week program in *Beyond Pritikin* nearly two decades ago and then brought out a more extensive version of that diet in *The Fat Flush Plan*, I helped revolutionize weight loss by introducing the concept of detox to the diet world. Years before Atkins, South Beach, and the Zone, I predicted that the low-fat, high-carb diets so popular in the 1980s were actually creating weight gain, sugar cravings, fatigue, and diabetes—health concerns that have taken on epidemic proportions today. I was the first to point out the importance of the essential fatty acids for weight loss as well as for overall health and beauty, a recurring theme in my two dozen books. My millions of readers around the world, and the millions more who visit my Web site (www.fasttrackdetox.com), have always known that they can count on me for sound, well-researched nutritional advice based on both real-life experience and scientific evidence.

Then, in November 2003, *Woman's World* magazine came to me with an unusual request. They wanted a one-day juice fast, the recipe for a special brew that would enable readers to quickly lose 3 to 5 pounds so they could fit into that special outfit or take off that holiday weight.

A fast can be a terrific weight-loss method because during a fast, the primary source of fuel for the cells is fat. Of course, I'd known for years that an improperly done fast can actually sabotage weight loss by disrupting your metabolism. The wrong kind of fasting can also threaten your health by stressing your liver, clogging your colon, and flooding your bloodstream with the oil-soluble toxins that your body had been storing in its fat.

On the other hand, a fast done right—with your body prepared for fasting and properly supported during the regime—can flush the accumulated toxins from your cells, accelerate your weight loss, cleanse your body, and combat the effects of aging. Periodic fasting of this type can clear up skin conditions, boost your energy, and put a sparkle in your eyes.

Moreover, a properly done fast offers you a chance to detoxify your body. A body overloaded with toxins and pollutants suffers from a weakened immune system, a stressed-out liver, and, in all probability, a malfunctioning colon. Such "toxic" bodies are far more vulnerable to disorders great and small, ranging from colds, flu, and fatigue to arthritis, asthma, and allergies—all the way up to autoimmune conditions, heart disease, and cancer. In other words, *properly done fasting is the missing link to better health.*

And fasting and detox have one more benefit, perhaps the most dramatic and the least well-known of all. *Fasting is the missing link to long-term weight loss.* That's because detox and weight loss go hand in hand. So the more toxic your body becomes, the more difficulty you will have losing weight and keeping it off.

Weight Loss and Toxicity: The Missing Link

The connection between weight loss and toxicity is so important, I'll say it again: *The more toxic your body becomes, the more difficulty you'll have losing weight.* Does that sound like an extreme statement? Then consider for a moment the "obesity epidemic" that you've no doubt read about. We now know that more than sixty diseases have been linked to obesity. More than 60 percent of Americans are overweight, while at least 30 percent of U.S. adults are obese—and close to 20 million children. Think of it—a whopping six out of ten Americans face a weight gain that might literally kill them by setting them up for diabetes, heart disease, and other deadly conditions.

Now recall the almost daily warnings about the growing amount of pollutants, toxins, and synthetic chemicals in our food, water, and air. The use of pesticides alone has doubled every ten years since 1945. Every day, corporations, cars, and homes release 700,000 tons of pollution into our air. Farmers spray seventy-two different pesticides on our fruits and veggies. Our cows and sheep are injected with estrogens to fatten them up and then stuffed with pesticide-laden grains to satisfy their artificial hunger.

Well, I'm here to tell you that there's a connection. Based on my twenty years as a practicing nutritionist, I see a clear link between rising levels of obesity and the fact that most of us are becoming more toxic every year.

1. **Our bodies are staggering under the enormous load of industrial toxins that have entered our food, water, and environment—and these toxins are making us fat.** First, we ingest the hormone-laden foods meant to fatten up cattle and sheep for market. Then our hormones are further disrupted by the pesticides, chemical fertilizers, and heavy metals that these poor animals consume with their feed. Finally, our poor polluted planet bombards us with new toxic invaders every day, from the methyl mercury in our fish, to the solvents in our acrylic nails, to the rocket fuel, of all things, that has seeped into the groundwater of twenty-two states. These toxins are in our homes, our workplace, our cosmetics, and our food. They're deadly to our health and disastrous for our weight.

2. **Most of us eat far less fiber than we need and consume far more sugar, refined flour, saturated fats, and protein than we should.** In this toxic era, we need fiber more than ever, to help us neutralize the toxins and scrub them out of our system. A diet rich in whole grains, legumes, fruits, and fresh vegetables

offers us plenty of fiber—but how many of us eat that way? We're more likely to consume fatty, sugary, and floury foods or to go on the low-carb, low-fiber diets like Atkins and South Beach. Previous generations of Americans ate twenty to thirty grams of fiber per day. Our current average has dropped to less than twelve. So the food we eat sits in our colons for weeks, months, even years, where it slowly putrefies, bloating our stomachs and poisoning our bodies. Our poor, overloaded livers are supposed to detoxify our bodies, but they can't keep up with this toxic challenge. They do the best they can, but how can they properly metabolize fat when they're assaulted by this daily dose of toxins? Once again, we gain weight.

3. **Low-carb diets are adding new stresses to our liver, colon, and entire digestive system.** Some people can lose weight on low-carb diets—I'll be the first to admit it. But the long-term consequences of low-carb diets can be disastrous for both health and long-term weight loss. First, low-carb diets like Atkins and South Beach steer dieters toward high-protein foods like beef, chicken, fish, and pork—the very foods simply loaded with the toxins we've just discussed. Then they urge dieters to avoid the fiber-rich fruits and vegetables that might help purify and eliminate those toxins. Finally, they load us up with so many proteins that we can't produce enough stomach acid to digest them all. Stress, vitamin and mineral deficiencies, and poor eating habits have already deprived most Americans of the stomach acid we need. So we end up with an acid reflux epidemic while the undigested meat and cheese rots right there in our gut, overloading our liver and intestines with such poisons as indican, ammonia, cadaverine, and histidine. And—you guessed it—our weight continues to rise.

Clearly, we Americans are sorely in need of both *diet and detox*—a safe, effective way to lose weight based on supporting our livers and colons. Maybe, I thought, the one-day weight-loss miracle that *Woman's World* had requested would allow me to kill two birds with one stone. With the right fast, dieters could lose significant amounts of weight virtually overnight, and they could also take advantage of fasting's age-old ability to cleanse and purify our bodies. A one-day fast would give both men and women a sense of how satisfying good nutrition and cellular cleansing can be. People who successfully completed a properly done fast might even move on to long-term lifestyle changes.

The key would be to develop a fast that provided dieters with adequate nutritional support, particularly for their livers and colons— our major detox organs. So I drew on my years of research, writing, and counseling to come up with a plan. The results were astounding.

The One-Day Detox Diet: A Proven System

First, the one-day fast I developed did indeed achieve immediate weight-loss results. *Woman's World* readers reported losing 3, 4, even 5 pounds in a single day. The special "miracle juice" I created for dieters to drink while they fasted successfully staved off hunger pangs, maintained metabolism, and provided the nutritional backup fasters need to support their livers and colons.

But my fast went far beyond simple weight loss. It also allowed dieters to taste the delights of detox, the enormous health benefits we can achieve by ridding our bodies of the toxins that bog them down.

Sure enough, the first people who tried my fast reported quick weight loss, no hunger, and vastly increased energy. As they told *Woman's World*:

> *My stomach wasn't bloated anymore. Within a few hours of starting, a friend told me my face looked thinner.*
> —JACKIE NEAL, THIRTY-TWO; LOST 3.5 POUNDS

> *Now my favorite black pants are loose in the waist and hips. I've never had results like this before!*
> —MAUREEN MACARTHUR,
> THIRTY-SIX, A MOTHER OF THREE; LOST 4 POUNDS

The day I did it, I was wearing a pair of drawstring pants. By
the end of the day, they were practically falling off . . . I did it
on the weekend, when I normally sit around and watch TV.
Instead, I cleaned my whole apartment.

—ANASTASIA SIGNORETTA,
TWENTY-SEVEN; LOST 3.5 POUNDS

Thrilled by these responses, I posted the *Woman's World* article on my Web site (www.annlouise.com), where it's not unusual to get more than 30,000 visitors in a single day. Suddenly, I was deluged with feedback. Dozens of dieters wrote me about their success on the one-day program, how they were losing pounds gained during travel or the holidays, how they could finally fit into that special size 8 dress or skinny pantsuit, how they were breaking through their dieting plateaus. They told me they felt lighter, cleaner, more energized. Some of them even told me they had started having better sex!

I heard both from my veteran Fat Flushers who wanted to shed some extra weight and from new dieters looking to ease into a healthier lifestyle. Some of the newbies told me that, indeed, my One-Day Diet had enabled them to make a new commitment to healthy eating for the first time in their lives, thanks to these impressive, instant results.

Here, I realized, was the opportunity I'd been seeking for a long time—a chance to combine my lifelong commitment to detoxification with an innovative approach to weight loss. Here was the next wave of health and healing, the missing link that could help women lose weight, regain their vitality, and glow with good health.

So I expanded the *Woman's World* plan, creating an entirely new way to combine weight loss and detox. This book is the result.

Losing Weight, Gaining Energy

As I started to come up with an improved and expanded version of Fast Track, I believed that my new plan would continue to offer the dramatic benefits that *Woman's World* readers had experienced with the earlier program. But like any good clinician, I wanted to test my hypothesis. So I shared this developing detox program with my own Fat Flushers as well as with more than 100 dieters in Syracuse, New York, under the guidance of a registered dietitian. The Syracuse group was composed of men and women ages sixteen to seventy, all of whom had struggled for a long time with weight loss and healthy eating.

And the program worked! In fact, the results were even better than my initial estimates, causing me to revise my prediction of the upper limit of one-day weight loss from 5 pounds to 8 pounds.

Most striking was the experience of Michael Pankhurst, a fifty-eight-year-old who had struggled with his weight throughout his life. Before starting the one-day fast, he pronounced himself "dubious." But by the end of the day, his doubts had vanished with his fat.

"I lost eight pounds," he enthused. "My mental clarity during the day was greatly improved. So was my energy level, despite a preexisting throat condition. And I wasn't even hungry. I think I will try to do it frequently, to boost mental clarity and weight loss."

As Michael discovered, the benefits of the One-Day Detox Diet went far beyond weight. Other dieters experienced the same lightness, energy, and mental clarity that the *Woman's World* dieters had felt. They also reported that the Fast Track got them back on track for healthy eating, enabled them to shed extra holiday and vacation pounds, and helped them break their dieting plateaus. They were impressed with their greater alertness, glowing skin, sparkling eyes, and toned, tight feeling. Many of them told me that they wanted to make the Fast Track a special ritual or a regular part of their routine—once a month or during the change of season—to regain that cleansed, energized feeling and sense of emotional and physical well-being. (And some of them, too, reported better sex after cleansing!)

I also noticed that some of the Syracuse fasters experienced some symptoms—headache, irritability, fatigue—that I knew resulted from caffeine addiction and insufficient liver support from their previous diet. With what I learned from their experience, I went on to design the expanded, fully supportive program that you see in this book.

The Fast Track: A Three-Stage Process

Thanks to my own clinical trials, I can assure you that the Fast Track is both an effective weight-loss plan and a superb detox system, a simple, easy, and effective way to lose weight and get your health back on the *fast* track.

What distinguishes the One-Day Detox Diet from all those other plans out there? Well, for one thing, although you will almost certainly lose between 3 and 8 pounds in a single day, you don't just subject your body to a fast unprepared. You spend an entire week on the Seven-Day Prequel, eating the Liver-Loving Foods that your body's major detox organ so desperately needs. You'll also load up on Colon-Caring Foods to help your colon purge the toxins and waste from your body.

Then, after the fast is over, you'll seal in the results with a Three-Day Sequel that includes liver and colon support along with special natural food sources of *probiotics*—fermented foods that support the friendly bacteria your system needs to synthesize vitamins and promote immune function. Finally, you'll learn about my Fast Track Detox Diet for Life, a clean, organic way of eating that includes all the foods and supplements you've consumed so far as well as two major new ones: *enzymes* and *nucleotides*. I consider these dietary elements to be among the major new frontiers in diet and nutritional health, and I'll tell you why in chapter 9.

So if you'd like to experience both immediate weight loss and long-term health, get on the *fast* track! You'll be amazed at what you can accomplish.

A Twenty-First-Century Caution

For centuries, people all over the world have taken advantage of fasting's near-miraculous benefits, making regular fasts and other detox procedures an integral part of their religious and cultural traditions. These practices included a wide range of fasting techniques, from "total" fasting to fasting that allowed water but no food products, to juice fasts and other severely restricted diets.

FAST TRACK: THE ONE-DAY DETOX DIET

Stage One: Seven-Day Prequel
Nourish yourself with Liver-Loving and Colon-Caring Foods to fortify your major detox and elimination organs during your one-day fast.

Stage Two: One-Day Fast
Fast for a single day while drinking a deliciously spiced Miracle Juice, specially designed to stave off hunger pangs, boost your metabolism, keep your blood sugar steady, and flush toxins from your system.

Stage Three: Three-Day Sequel
Ease back into eating with more Liver-Loving and Colon-Caring Foods to flush any remaining toxins from your system.
Consume foods rich in probiotics, which will support the friendly bacteria that keep your digestion and immune system working at peak efficiency.

FOR FAT FLUSHERS . . .

For those of you who either are on the Fat Flush Plan or were planning to start, don't worry! You can easily do the Fast Track while you are on any phase of the Fat Flush Plan, especially if you want more detox benefits or if you've plateaued. Just make sure you have completed at least one week of Phase 1. Then, during the three days after your fast, include the probiotics element from chapter 8 of this book into your current Fat Flush phase.

In the European tradition, Hippocrates, the founder of Western medicine, advocated periodic fasting as a way to cleanse the body and allow the digestive system to rest. Galen, the medieval physician who pioneered our understanding of the heart and circulatory system, both fasted himself and prescribed the approach to his patients. And Paracelsus, whose groundbreaking discoveries anticipated modern theories about germs and viruses, called fasting "the greatest remedy— the physician within."

Both Western and Eastern traditions have seen fasting and other means of detox as a way to combine spiritual and physical cleansing, simultaneously purifying body, mind, and spirit. Christianity, Judaism, Islam, Buddhism, Hinduism, and many African religions have employed fasting for a number of purposes: purification, penance, mourning, preparation for ceremonies, and to enhance one's own spiritual and mental powers.[1] In India, the ancient tradition of Ayurvedic medicine is based on freeing the body from toxins, which practitioners believe can help the individual's spiritual state as well. Perhaps as a result, fasting has been advocated by many yoga practitioners and spiritual teachers.

In North America, Native Americans turned to sweat lodges for both spiritual and bodily purification. The Finns, Swedes, and other Scandinavians sweated the winter blues away with steamy saunas. And many European physicians routinely prescribe fasting as an effective way to give our bodies a rest, to lighten our toxic load, and to allow stressed or overworked organs to repair themselves. It's only in the United States that the medical establishment has been so resistant to fasting and other types of detoxification.

So until the nineteenth century or so, fasting was a well-respected means of cleansing, purifying, and rejuvenating our bodies, minds, and spirits. Then came the modern industrial age. Suddenly our food, water, and air were burdened with thousands of industrial chemicals, additives, and pollutants. According to the U.S. Environmental Protection Agency (EPA), traces of toxic chemicals can now be found in nearly every single one of us—and guess where those toxins reside? That's right, in our fat. So when we lose weight quickly, as we do during a fast, those poisons and pollutants go right into our bloodstreams, putting us at risk for a whole host of diseases, including cancer, birth defects, and neuro-degenerative diseases such as Parkinson's.

Let's face it, we're living in a sea of chemicals, assaulted each day by poisons in our air, water, food, and homes. According to the EPA, in 1994, corporations released more than 2.2 billion pounds of toxic chemicals into our environment—and that figure has only increased with each passing year.

Don't count on escaping the toxins by staying indoors, either. In addition to the poisons we consume in our food and drink, indoor air pollution may well be ten times worse than the outdoor variety. We're assaulted by cleaning products, plastics, office supplies, pesticides, and synthetic fibers—even by scented beauty and hygiene products. The innocent-looking particleboard or plywood furniture we buy contains formaldehyde. So does our carpeting. Our homes are clearly no safe haven from a toxic world.[2]

"Well," you may be thinking, "it's highly unlikely that all these toxic substances have actually made their way into *my* body. After all, I live in a pretty clean area and I've always watched what I eat." Don't count on that, either. In 1999 and 2000, the Centers for Disease Control and Prevention (CDC) tested some 2,500 people for 116 chemicals. Every single person in the "body burden" study, no matter what their age, location, or lifestyle, tested positive for at least some environmental toxins.

To me, that's a frightening statistic. Whether we live in the heart of New York City, the suburbs of a Southern city, or the wilds of Wyoming, we're being exposed to poisons in our air, food, water, and homes. How can those poisons, which are lodged in our organs and bloodstream and fat cells, fail to affect our health?

As a matter of fact, few studies exist on the dangers of environmental toxins. Virtually all of the 80,000 industrial chemicals, additives, and preservatives currently in use were invented sometime within the last seventy-five years—most more recently than that—so we have very little scientific evidence on how dangerous they are.

However, cancer rates have risen from 20 to 50 percent since 1970, while the number of asthma sufferers has grown by 75 percent since 1980. Isn't it just common sense to suppose that this new incidence of disease may be related to environmental pollution? When you think about the scientific studies we do have on such toxins as Agent Orange, pesticides, mercury, and lead, why should we imagine that all the other heavy metals, insecticides, and industrial chemicals out there are safe for us and our children?[3]

Toxic Problems, Detox Solutions

If environmental toxins are the problem, you'd think detoxification would be the solution. But again, medical and scientific evidence is lacking. One of the most severe frustrations I've felt over the years is over the resistance the medical establishment has to acknowledging the benefits of detox. Although any physician would readily admit the need to pump a person's stomach to remove poison or to chelate lead from the blood of someone with lead poisoning, few conventional doctors take the logical next step—recognizing the need to remove *other* toxic elements from our bodies. Indeed, many doctors poohpooh the notion of detoxification so vigorously, you might think that scientific studies have actually shown it to be without value.

But the truth is not so simple. In fact, the scientific establishment has done virtually no research into detox at all, except where alcohol or drugs are concerned. Far from establishing that detoxification won't work, mainstream science has largely ignored the topic.

Of course, detox isn't the only subject medical science has failed to test. Did you realize that there are no double-blind studies on whether aspirin relieves headache? People simply started using it before the U.S. Food and Drug Administration (FDA) ever required testing. It seemed to work, so they kept using it. But there's no evidence that they should.

Likewise, there are no double-blind studies on coronary artery surgery. How could there be? A double-blind study requires that no one—neither doctor nor patient—know which group got the real treatment and which got the placebo. Doctors could hardly give coronary patients placebo surgery, so they simply use a treatment they know and trust. In fact, only 30 percent of medical procedures are supported by double-blind studies, but we'd never expect our physicians to stop using the other 70 percent.[4]

Fortunately, a few detox studies have been conducted, primarily by scientists committed to alternative medicine. A study reported in *Alternative Therapies in Health and Medicine* tested twenty-five otherwise healthy people before and then seven days after they'd undergone a liver detox program. Participants filled out questionnaires and underwent drug challenge tests, procedures whereby they were given small amounts of drugs, including caffeine, to see how quickly the liver could perform its detoxifying function of clearing the foreign substance from the bloodstream.

Based on a caffeine clearance test, subjects' liver detox capacities improved by 23 percent; based on the questionnaires, their liver functions rose by 47 percent. Lab tests also showed an improved ratio of sulfate to creatinine in the subjects' urine, a medical indicator that points to improved liver function. The researchers concluded, "Symptoms of poor health in people free from diagnosed disease may be related to toxic buildup,"[5] which certainly implies that reducing toxic buildup might improve our health.

If detoxification is so helpful to healthy individuals, how might it benefit those of us who are chronically ill? An earlier study in *Alternative Therapies* suggests that once again, detox can make a dramatic difference in our health. For ten weeks, twenty-two chronically ill participants in the study were given a special diet, while eighty-four subjects were given that diet along with a detox program. Both groups did better on the diet, but the detox group's progress was markedly better, showing a 52 percent reduction in symptoms, compared to only 22 percent in the control group. The detox patients likewise enjoyed improved liver functions, increased sulfate-to-creatinine ratios, and better absorption of nutrients.[6]

The *Alternative Medicine Review* has likewise suggested that a toxic system has been associated with a number of chronic diseases, including chronic fatigue syndrome, fibromyalgia, Parkinson's disease, and cancer.[7] The conclusion seems obvious: Low-level toxicity is behind many of today's illnesses, which makes detoxing essential for our health.[8]

Although it's always dangerous to cite personal experience alongside scientific studies—after all, we all have our biases—I'd be irresponsible if I didn't add that in my twenty years of nutritional practice, I've witnessed numerous near-miracle cures of people suffering from toxicity whose health improved dramatically from detox programs. I've seen how many of my family members, friends, and patients have enjoyed remarkable benefits from fasting and detox.

I've also had my own personal chance to observe the benefits of internal cleansing. Although for years I recommended against water fasting and even against prolonged juice fasts, I've always practiced short-term juice fasts, in which the liver and colon get the proper support before, during, and after the fast. I do my own fasts at least three or four times a year, usually around the fall and spring equinoxes, and whenever I feel myself to be on overload, whether physically, mentally, or spiritually.

My own experience with fasting has convinced me of the myriad benefits of this ancient tradition. Fasting serves as a kind of sabbath on which I take a day of rest from eating but also from working—an essential aspect of healing for a workaholic like me! Fasting is my time to "be" instead of "do," and I put all work and household chores aside to focus on contemplation and journal writing. I've noticed over the years how wonderfully a fast day helps me slow down, clarifying my thinking even as my thoughts become more peaceful. For me, a fast day is a time for reflection on all areas of my life, a time to connect with my inner self. I always end my fasts feeling renewed, buoyed by the fresh sense of potential for my life.

And, of course, fasting helps jump-start your weight loss! Properly done fasting not only frees us from the fattening toxins that overload our environment but is also a quick, safe, and easy way to break through our dieting plateaus; to overcome the weight gain that often follows vacations and holidays; or to get ourselves back on track when we've found ourselves overindulging in sweets, starches, or other unhealthy foods. Just make sure you follow the protocol: the Seven-Day

Prequel (chapter 5) (or one week of Fat Flush Phase 1), the One-Day Detox Diet (chapter 6), and the Three-Day Sequel (chapter 8). Otherwise, what started out as a weight-loss and health benefit could end up having just the opposite effect.

Fasting for Health and Weight Loss

When we begin to detoxify, whether through fasting or another means (such as Phase 1 of the Fat Flush Plan), two simultaneous procedures begin. One takes place on the cellular level, as each of our body's cells gets an opportunity to release any toxins it may hold. That's why drinking lots of fluids is such an important part of any fast—it helps flush out these toxins as they are released into the bloodstream.

At the same time, our organs have an extra chance to eliminate toxins stored inside the body but outside the cells. Fecal matter that has clogged the colon, for example, or mucus that has blocked the lungs, may be released. We may urinate or defecate more than usual or we may find ourselves sweating, coughing, or experiencing other symptoms of our body's new determination to unload the poisons it has stored for so long.

Although this so-called healing crisis can be uncomfortable for some people, a good detox makes us feel much better in the end. And no wonder! Our bodies are finally shedding the poisons that have clogged and overloaded them. According to my personal friend and longtime detox practitioner Elson Haas, M.D., you can expect numerous physical, mental, and spiritual benefits from undergoing an effective detox:[9]

Increased energy	Self-confidence
Anti-aging effects	Greater motivation and optimism
Clearer skin	
Sharpened senses (vision, hearing, taste)	A sense of personal beauty
	More restful sleep
A cleaner personal space	Help in changing habits

Increased relaxation

More creativity and inspiration

Fewer or less severe allergies

Improved mental and emotional clarity

Improved personal organization

Long-term changes in diet

Some experts also believe that fasting and detox can help us overcome food cravings and other addictions, helping us regain our natural hunger and restoring our innate appreciation for the taste, smell, and texture of food. Because my Fast Track provides special nutritional support for our hardworking liver and colon, you can add better liver function, improved elimination, and an increased sense of well-being to the list of benefits.

Protecting Our Planet

I know the major reason you're reading this book is because you're interested in losing weight and boosting your health. But I can't end this first chapter without pointing out another benefit of fasting—the boost in awareness that it creates not only of our bodies, minds, and spirits but also of this beautiful planet on which we all depend. Every day, I read new reports of pesticides, toxins, insecticides, and industrial chemicals making their way into our bodies. But these poisons not only are hurting our health but are also affecting farm animals, wild creatures, our lakes and rivers and oceans, our groundwater and soil, the very air we breathe. What kind of legacy are we leaving for future generations? What kind of future are we building for ourselves? My hope is that each of you who reads this book and undertakes a personal detox will spend at least some of your fasting day thinking about our wonderful planet and how we can help it, too, cleanse itself of the toxins we have created and help protect it for the future.

Using This Book

For nearly a quarter of a century, I've been helping men and women learn more about their bodies, with a particular focus on detox and cleansing. Although I'm best known for my weight-loss books, my true love has always been detox, to the point that—I'll admit it—some of my colleagues call me "the Colon Queen." Detox and cleansing were my first love as a nutritionist, and they've remained my passion all these years, all the more so because I've come to see that they're crucial to weight loss as well as to health.

So when it came time to write this book, I couldn't resist sharing with you the wonderful information I've gathered over the years, offering you the building blocks to become your own nutritionist and your own detox specialist. That's why, as you read on, you'll find chapters on environmental toxins (chapter 2), on the dangers of low-carb dieting (chapter 3), and on your major detox organs—the liver and the colon (chapter 4). I firmly believe that if you know what's going on in your body, you'll follow the One-Day Detox Diet more effectively, along with every element of the Seven-Day Prequel and the Three-Day Sequel.

But I also know that some people prefer taking action right away. So for those of you eager to get right to the diet, go ahead and turn to chapter 5, "Getting Ready." That first week of liver and colon preparation is *essential* to the success of the One-Day Detox Diet, so you can't skip that. If you do, you risk health problems, unpleasant symptoms, and the likelihood of gaining back all the weight you lose during your fast. But you don't *have* to read chapters 2, 3, and 4—they're optional.

I sincerely hope, however, that you do read those chapters. I'd love to share with you all the insight and knowledge I've gained from my years doing research and working with clients and dieters around the country. The choice is yours; either way, I'm thrilled you're giving the Fast Track a try. All you have to lose is a few pounds and all those toxins that are dragging you down. All you have to gain is a whole new way of life.

The release from all that buildup is amazing!! I finally feel like I have my body back and not some alien living in it.
—BONITA JEAN MANION, FIFTY; LOST 2.5 POUNDS

Why You Need This Book

*Man is more the product of his environment
than of his genetic endowment.*
—Rene Jules Dubos

I'll never forget it.

I was giving a workshop for the Learning Annex in San Francisco when I made what I thought was an offhand reference to the relationship between weight loss and the environment.

"Of course, living in a toxic world is probably our biggest single obstacle to losing weight," I told this group of veteran dieters, many of whom were there precisely because they expected me to offer some new suggestions for the weight loss they'd struggled with for so many frustrating years. "When our bodies are assaulted by so many pesticides, petroleum-based fertilizers, additives, preservatives, antibiotics, hormones, and environmental pollutants, that's bad for our health, of course—but it also makes it much harder to lose weight and keep it off."

I was about to move on to my next point when I was interrupted by a sea of waving hands. "Wait just a minute," said one woman in her late twenties, who later told me she'd been a runner, and a dieter, since her teenage years. "I know pollution is bad for our bodies in general, sure, everybody knows that. But how does it affect our weight?" The emphatically nodding heads across the room told me that she was far from the only dieter puzzled about this connection.

Well, I told her, the liver is your body's filter, charged with neutralizing all sorts of substances from the waste products of everyday metabolism to the ever-increasing load of toxins from our air, water, food, cosmetics, and workplace. One of the most serious results of an overstressed or toxic liver is that it becomes so bogged down, it can't fully metabolize fat. As a result, it dumps fat and cholesterol back into the bloodstream, sabotaging your weight loss and putting you at risk for numerous health problems, including indigestion, fatigue, high cholesterol, depression, mood swings, lupus, arthritis, and other autoimmune conditions. A toxic liver also creates disastrous results for your skin, leaving you with a tendency to blotchy patches and rashes.

Meanwhile, your colon—designed to eliminate both natural bodily waste and toxins—is likewise laboring under a double strain. If you're not getting enough fiber, and most Americans aren't, especially if they're on a low-carb diet, your colon doesn't have the support it needs to do its job. An overworked colon means that toxins and bile (a crucial substance produced by the liver) can sit in your gut too long. Eventually, your body reabsorbs the toxins and sends them back to the liver once again.

"And that's just the health side of the picture," I told my increasingly spellbound listeners. "I can also tell you that wastes left in the colon can harden and create impactions that cause the colon to expand, resulting in added pounds and inches to your abdominal area. That's not fat, it's leftover food and waste products."

In other words, I concluded, a toxic liver and a clogged colon will sabotage a healthy eating plan faster than a double-dip ice-cream cone! What's the point of struggling to manage our food intake if our organs are giving way under the strain of processing a toxic overload?

Now the interruption came from an older woman's insistently waving hand. She looked to be in her mid-forties, a tall, striking woman who seemed tired and discouraged. Although I could see that she'd worked hard at keeping her weight down, I was struck by her blotchy skin and the dark circles around her eyes. Her scale might be giving her the answers she wanted, but her mirror definitely wasn't.

"How do we know if toxins are our problem?" she asked breath-lessly, and again, her neighbors nodded. "Because I'll tell you, I eat lots of fruits and veggies, so I know I'm getting my fiber. I've given up sugar, except maybe once or twice a week. I'm not on any medica-tions, and I drink a few glasses of wine a month, at most. But I'm still having trouble keeping the weight off. And I'm tired all the time."

I ended up meeting with this woman privately and helping her identify the toxins lurking in her diet and her environment: the pesticide-laden strawberries she had each morning for breakfast, the mercury-ridden fish she had been so good about eating five times a week, the hidden toxins in her cosmetics, and the mercury in her fill-ings. Although not everyone is equally sensitive to these toxic triggers, this woman was—and you may be, too. I told her about some rela-tively simple ways of detoxing her body, her diet, and her home, tech-niques that I'll share with you throughout this book.

But first things first. By now you're probably wondering if you, too, are suffering from toxic overload that is sabotaging your weight loss, masking your natural beauty, and threatening your health. Luckily for us, the body never lies. Once you learn how to read the clues your body is giving you, you can take the necessary steps through the Fast Track to find natural and nonprescription solutions for those symptoms that concern you the most.

Read Your Body Like a Book: Signs of Distress

1. Do you have . . .

   . . . acne, blemishes, hives, or itchy rashes?

   . . . discoloration in the eyes?

   . . . red, swollen, or teary eyes?

   . . . hemorrhoids or varicose veins?

   . . . hormonal imbalances such as PMS, menstrual problems, or menopausal concerns, particularly hot flashes?

. . . heat in the upper body, such as warm face or hot eyes?

. . . light-colored stools?

. . . gas, bloating, belching, and nausea, especially after eating fatty foods?

. . . difficulty digesting fats?

. . . mild frontal headaches after fatty meals?

. . . tendency to loss of appetite or eating disorder?

. . . weight gain, particularly when you are controlling your food intake?

. . . feelings of tiredness or sleepiness after eating?

. . . tendency to wake between 1 A.M. and 3 A.M.?

. . . weak tendons, ligaments, or muscles?

. . . pain under the right shoulder blade?

. . . excessive, unexplained, or sudden bursts of anger, irritability, or rage?

. . . depression, particularly depression unrelated or disproportionate to life events?

. . . elevated liver enzymes (SGOT, SGPT)?

. . . high bilibrubin levels?

✴ Regardless of whether you have one or ten of these symptoms, your body is trying to give you an SOS. Whether your symptoms are PMS, discolored stools, waking up between 1 A.M. and 3 A.M., or any of the other symptoms, your capacity to detox may be impaired and you may be suffering from a sluggish or toxic liver. You will definitely need to build up your liver before the One-Day Detox Diet and support your liver after the fast, so don't skip the Seven-Day Prequel or the Three-Day Sequel, both of which include a nutritional strategy for a healthy liver.

2. Do you have . . .

. . . bad breath or an offensive body odor?

. . . a frequent bitter taste in your mouth?

. . . a coated tongue?

. . . putrid and/or painful gas?

. . . digestive disorders?

. . . problems with elimination?

. . . constipation or diarrhea?

. . . long, thin, or foul-smelling stools; stools with undigested food particles?

. . . lower back pain?

. . . abdominal discomfort or fullness?

. . . rectal itching?

. . . bruises that don't heal?

. . . difficulty perspiring?

. . . joint aches and pains?

. . . arthritis?

. . . colitis or diverticulitis?

. . . systematic yeast infections or problems with *Candida*?

. . . parasites or worms?

. . . multiple allergic response syndrome (MARS)?

. . . multiple food allergies or sensitivities to the environment (perfumes, other fragrances, car fumes or other odors)?

✷ Again, your body is sending you a cry for help with even one of these symptoms, which could indicate impaired elimination and a toxic or sluggish colon. Whether your symptoms are a coated tongue, constipation, *Candida* infection, or any of the other symptoms, you will definitely need to stimulate your ability to eliminate waste, so don't skip the Seven-Day Prequel or the Three-Day Sequel, both of which include a nutritional strategy for a healthy colon.

Warning: Toxic Signs Ahead

In addition to the symptoms we've just listed, you might notice many other signs of toxic overload that indicate the need for the One-Day Detox Diet:

- Frequent coughs

- Stuffy nose

- Sinus problems

- A tendency to colds and flu

- Exhaustion, lethargy, and fatigue

- Mental dullness or poor memory

- Premature aging

And if you have trouble losing weight or maintaining your ideal weight, even when you regulate your food intake and exercise regularly, you should definitely consider whether a toxic liver or colon is part of the problem.[1]

Now, if you've taken this quiz and are feeling a bit overwhelmed by the results, don't despair. The bad news is the extent to which toxic substances in our food, air, water, and environment are damaging our health and sabotaging our weight loss. But the good news is how much we can do about it. By undertaking the Seven-Day Prequel, One-Day Detox Diet, and Three-Day Sequel, laid out in chapters 5, 6, and 8, you can start right away to support your system and help your body eliminate that toxic buildup. And by following the suggestions for lifelong health in chapter 9, you can stay on the Fast Track and even move on to the next level of lifelong weight control, beauty, and vibrant health.

I firmly believe that the Fast Track One-Day Detox Diet represents the next wave in healthy weight loss. Reducing your body's chemical burden; supporting its primary detoxifiers, the liver and the colon; and choosing organic and other clean foods is no longer a luxury but a necessity. It's crystal clear that diet plus detox is the coming trend, simply because toxins are taxing our weight as well as our health.

Now, at this point, you've got two choices. If, like me, you enjoy knowing what's going on in your body and want to learn more about how toxins, additives, and preservatives are affecting you, read on. You might be particularly interested if you've been having any of the symptoms you just read about, because toxins in your liver and colon may just be part of the problem. In this chapter, I'll tell you about the heavy metals, pesticides, "false estrogens," and other environmental dangers that are giving you symptoms and making you fat. In chapter 3, I'll show you how low-carb diets may have been making your system even more toxic, and I'll tell you about two major hidden health threats—low stomach acid and excessive gluten—that are currently threatening many of us. In chapter 4, I'll give you a quick tour of your major detox organs, the liver and the colon, so you can see for yourself how toxins weigh your body down.

But you do have another choice. If you'd like to jump straight to the solution, move right on to chapter 5, which will tell you how to begin preparing for your detox experience. After a week of eating the Liver-Loving and Colon-Caring Foods listed in that chapter, you'll be all set for the One-Day Detox Diet described in chapter 6, followed up by the Three-Day Sequel in chapter 8, which will really help you seal in the results.

The choice is yours, although I personally advise you to keep on reading so that you get the big picture about the toxins that assault your body every day. After all, you need to know your enemy before you can defeat it.

The Body Burden

Recently a number of research organizations sponsored a fascinating, and disturbing, study. The Mount Sinai School of Medicine in New York, the Environmental Working Group, and a research institute known as Commonweal wanted to discover the "body burden"—the load of toxic chemicals—that affects each of our bodies. So they recruited a high-profile group of volunteers, including journalist Bill Moyers, who agreed to be tested for a wide range of environmental pollutants.

The results, as reported by environmentalist Alexandra Rome in a March 28, 2004, article in the *San Francisco Chronicle*, were deeply troubling. Rome, herself a participant in the study, discovered that her body had measurable levels of eighty-six toxic chemicals, including twenty-seven different versions of polychlorinated biphenyls (PCBs) and dioxins. This last finding was especially disturbing, considering that the manufacture of PCBs was banned in the United States in 1976.

Even more upsetting to Rome was the realization that she had been tested for only 210 of the more than 80,000 chemicals licensed for commercial use. Clearly, Rome wrote, she—and the rest of us— have stored far more manufactured chemicals than these test results revealed.

Moreover, since most of these chemicals have come into use only within the last 75 years, we actually know very little about how they affect us. As a result, Rome added with more than a touch of sarcasm, our bodies have become "part of a vast chemistry experiment."

As Rome went on to explain in her article, the number of industrial chemicals licensed for commercial use is growing rapidly each year. In addition to the 80,000 already licensed, an additional 2,000 new synthetic chemicals make their way into the marketplace each year. Thus, in 1998, U.S. industries produced 6.5 trillion pounds of some 9,000 different chemicals. But in 2000, major U.S. companies released 7.1 billion pounds of 650 chemicals into our environment— a figure that doesn't even take into account the additional activities of small companies.

Rome was particularly shocked at her own test results because she'd spent her life working on environmental and health issues. Such heightened awareness, she'd thought, should have protected her from environmental dangers. No such luck.

"I had secretly harbored the hope that I would find I didn't have much of the bad stuff in me," she wrote in her *San Francisco Chronicle* account. "After all, I have been privileged to live a 'clean' life. I haven't worked in factories or lived in heavily industrial areas; I've had access to good, organic food; I'm well educated and knowledgeable about the dangers of pesticides."

However, Rome wrote, *"we are all in this chemical soup together. Chemicals in our environment don't discriminate"* (emphasis added).

In her moving, first-person article, Rome went on to detail her own history of autoimmune disease, fibromyalgia, a rare cardiac syndrome, and a breast condition generally considered a precursor to breast cancer. Getting her "body burden" test results made her wonder how environmental toxins had affected her health—and how they might affect the health of her children.

Once you know about the body burden, you see signs everywhere of the numerous toxins we're exposed to every day. For example, here are thirteen heavy metals to which we have daily exposure: lead, mercury, cadmium, cobalt, antinomy, barium, beryllium, cesium, molybdenum, platinum, thallium, tungsten, and uranium. In addition, we come into daily contact with the cotinine in tobacco smoke, at least six different types of pesticides, and seven different types of plastic whose molecules migrate into our food.[2]

In my book *How to Stay Young and Healthy in a Toxic World*, I identified the most prevalent toxic invaders and showed how to eliminate them from our lives. Since that time, my friend Stephen Sinatra, M.D., fellow of the American College of Cardiology and of the American College of Nutrition, has become a champion of raising public awareness about the dangers that lurk in the environment. In the March 2003 edition of his newsletter, *The Sinatra Health Report*, he offered his own hit list of twenty toxins found in everyday life, which I for one find enlightening—and downright scary:

- Insecticide residues: organic rotenone

- Prescription drugs: acetaminophen (Tylenol), aspirin, and nonsteroidal anti-inflammatory drugs (NSAIDs)

- Alcohol

- Indoor and outdoor air pollution

- Cigarette smoke

- Formaldehyde (in our new carpets, in processed wood furniture, and from mice)

- Soft drinks (loaded with phosphoric acid)

- Trans fatty acids (found in fast foods)

- Char-broiled meats (loaded with carcinogens)

- Hair dyes, cosmetics, and deodorants

- Petrochemicals, including xenobiotics and xenoestrogens (synthetic estrogens or estrogen mimics)

- Heavy metals: iron, copper, mercury, lead

- Processed meats (loaded with nitrites)

- Radon

- Gasoline

- Chlorinated water (which some researchers have predicted may be the greatest threat to our immune system in the next two decades, since chlorine kills lactobacilli, the "friendly bacteria" in our gut that combat harmful bacteria)

- Toxic fish (loaded with methyl mercury)

- Perchlorate (rocket fuel that leaks into our water supply)

- Industrial chemicals found in home cleaning fluids

- Phthalates (new varieties of plastics)[3]

These everyday toxins are everywhere—in our food, air, water; at home and at work; in the city and in the country. In fact, let me take you on a tour of the environmental poisons we encounter every day:[4]

- **Air** is polluted with chemicals from industrial activity; automobiles; cigarette smoke; and numerous indoor sources, including scented beauty and hygiene products, cleaning products, synthetic fibers, plastics, office supplies, plywood, particleboard, gas appliances, and even wallpaper.

- **Water** absorbs the chemicals that make their way into our rivers and streams as well as pollutants that soak into our groundwater. The EPA has discovered that more than 55,000 chemical dump holes currently exist—each one a potential source of leakage into our groundwater. Chemical fertilizers add their polluting effects, while the chlorine added to our drinking water—a key protection against typhoid, dysentery, and similar diseases—may combine with certain substances to form carcinogenic hydrocarbons. Even if you drink only filtered or bottled water, you're not off the hook, since 50 to 70 percent of adult exposure to waterborne pollutants comes in our bath or shower.

- **Food** is contaminated by chemical fertilizers, pesticides, polluted groundwater, additives, plastic packaging, leaded cans, and aluminum containers. Imported foods carry the extra whammy of pesticides, including DDT, banned in the United States but not abroad. Fish are increasingly polluted with mercury. And, as Rome discovered, highly toxic PCBs continue to lurk in our food, air, and water, despite the 1976 ban on their manufacture.

  D. Lindsey Berkson, a bioenvironmentalist educated at Tulane University, adds a chilling note in her book *Hormone Deception,* in which she cites a shocking Associated Press story. It seems that toxic heavy metals, such as cadmium, lead, and arsenic, along with dioxins and perhaps even radioactive waste, are routinely used to fertilize our fields. In Gore, Oklahoma, for example, low-level radioactive waste from a nearby uranium-processing plant is licensed as a commercial fertilizer and sprayed over 9,000 acres of grazing land, where it presumably makes its way into the live-stock that munch on the newly fertilized grass. Although many other industrialized nations regulate the use of fertilizers, the United States does not, which means that medical, municipal, and industrial waste can all be spread over the ground where our crops grow and our cattle graze. Municipal sewage systems alone, says Berkson, sell some 36 percent of their 11.6 billion pounds of waste materials to farmers looking for fertilizer.[5]

No Diet Without Detox

If you've experienced any of the health problems I described in the quiz earlier in this chapter, you may already suspect a link between pollution and your health. But even if you've been feeling strong and healthy, you should be aware that, like Rome and the others in her study, you've almost certainly absorbed an enormous body burden of toxins, most of which are stored in your fat.

That brings me to a profound irony. Many of us decide to lose weight precisely because we value our health. Yet losing excess weight can actually weaken our defenses against these deadly chemicals. As our fat melts away, it releases the toxins that have been stored there, putting us at risk for new health problems, even as losing weight solves some of the old ones.

That's why I believe our twenty-first-century slogan must be "No Diet Without Detox!" Finding a way to cleanse our bodies of the toxins that flood our environment is crucial for all of us, and even more urgent for those of us who are losing weight. Otherwise, we're not only at the mercy of toxins in our environment but, by going on our diets and losing weight, also literally poisoning ourselves.

Are Chemicals Making You Fat?

We've already seen how environmental toxins overstress our livers and colons, making it harder for our bodies to metabolize fat and digest food. In chapter 4, we'll learn even more about how these vital organs affect our weight loss. But beyond the effect on our liver and colon, environmental toxins have a much more insidious ability to sabotage our weight.

Many scientists believe that the human body, when working properly, has a built-in weight-regulation system, the result of a complicated interaction among hormones, organs, calories, and physical activity. All things being equal, we should feel hungry when we need food, and full when we're nourished. Our natural appetite should regulate itself to ensure that our weight stays at a stable, healthy level.

Sadly, all things are *not* equal. New scientific evidence now suggests that many environmental toxins, in addition to poisoning our bodies, behave as though they were specifically intended to disrupt our natural weight-regulation system.

In some cases, this is literally true. The feed that nonorganic farmers give to their cows, lambs, pigs, chickens, and turkeys is deliberately designed to cause those animals to gain weight, fattening them up for the marketplace. When we consume the meat and dairy products that come from those animals, we start "fattening up," too.

However, even industrial chemicals intended to kill insects, preserve wood, or protect crops from fungus seem to have this fattening effect, disrupting our natural weight regulation and making us vulnerable to weight gain. Although most industrial chemicals have not been specifically studied for their weight-gain effects, virtually every study that has been done seems to point in this direction.

One of the pioneers in the field of "fattening chemicals" is Paula Baillie-Hamilton, M.D., a British specialist in human metabolism and environmental health. Baillie-Hamilton has published an extensive study of the numerous synthetic chemicals currently pervading our environment. The conclusion she drew was nothing short of remarkable.

"In plain English," she writes, "I discovered that these chemicals appear to be making us fat . . . Time and again, when I learned about a different group of pesticides or environmental pollutants, I would soon discover that they too could cause weight gain."[6]

Baillie-Hamilton explains that there are two types of fattening chemicals in our environment. There are the chemicals that farmers add to their feed specifically to fatten up their livestock and to alter their animals' metabolism.[7] And there are also the pesticides, medicines, heavy metals, synthetic materials, solvents, environmental pollutants, fire retardants, and thousands of other substances that flood our environment.[8] Even though this second group of chemicals wasn't invented for the purpose of making anyone fat, that seems to be the effect they have. By disrupting the natural weight regulation built into our metabolism, this second group of chemicals makes it harder for us to know when we're hungry, when we need to keep eating, and how much we need to move to use up the calories we've taken in.

There is further evidence for linking the plethora of synthetic chemicals in our environment to the emerging obesity epidemic.[9] Between 1930 and 2000, the number of synthetic chemicals in use skyrocketed—and so did the number of overweight adults in the United States. Here are just two of many animal studies suggesting that chemicals are disrupting our metabolism and helping make us fat.

In one experiment, mice were exposed to dieldrin, an insecticide used from the 1950s to protect cotton, corn, and citrus crops; to exterminate mosquitoes; and to preserve wood. Although dieldrin has been banned for nearly all uses in the United States since 1985, it is still present in our environment in high levels, according to the Children's Health Environment Coalition, particularly because it also exists as the result of the breakdown of another insecticide, aldrin, which was used in the United States for termite control until 1987.

You might think that a poison designed to kill bugs wouldn't affect a mouse's weight one way or the other. But in fact, the dieldrin-treated mice more than doubled their total body fat.[10]

In a similar study, animals were treated with hexachlorobenzene (HCB), a substance used in making rubber, dyes, and wood preservatives as well as for treating fungus in wheat. The HCB-dosed animals gained significantly more weight than their untreated counterparts, even though they were fed 50 percent less food than the HCB-free animals.[11]

Given the effects of the fattening pesticides, pollutants, and other toxins in our environment, why aren't we all obese? According to

Baillie-Hamilton, genetics, individual eating habits, variations in our exposure to chemicals, and age all play a role in our actual weight, as does getting the proper nutrients and regular exercise. It's encouraging to know that even under the assault of fattening chemicals, there's still plenty we can do to keep our weight down.

But, Baillie-Hamilton points out, the problem underlying our obesity epidemic is that most people's natural ability to regulate their weight is being disrupted. Both the constant assault of toxic chemicals and a lack of the nutrients we need is making us fat.[12]

I would add that those of us who support our liver and colon have an enormous advantage in the weight-loss battle, because these organs are crucial in the effort to rid our bodies of fattening chemicals. That's why detox and cleansing are at the heart of my Fast Track. The Seven-Day Prequel and Three-Day Sequel will ensure that you get the nutrients you need, while the One-Day Detox Diet will start to flush the toxins from your body. Then you can take detox and cleansing to the next level by following the suggestions in chapter 9.

Xenoestrogens: False Friends, Indeed!

One theory about why the chemicals cited by Baillie-Hamilton are inducing weight gain has to do with the way they mimic the effects of estrogen in our bodies. That's why this group of toxins has come to be known as "false estrogens," or *xenoestrogens*. These poisonous infiltrators, whose use has skyrocketed since World War II, find various ways of inducing, blocking, or otherwise scrambling our hormonal signals, either because they have deliberately been intended to do so (as in weight-inducing animal feeds) or as an accidental effect of what happens as they break down (as in the experiments when animals were given dieldrin or HCB). Either way, xenoestrogens are contributing to a relatively new condition known as *estrogen dominance*—one symptom of which is a tendency to gain weight.

Estrogen, of course, is the female hormone connected to such vital female functions as menstruation, pregnancy, and menopause. Estrogen tends to stimulate cell growth, signaling our bodies to build up uterine tissue every month, for example, or helping our ovaries instruct one egg each month to mature. In men, estrogen also promotes cell growth, healing, and other vital functions.

The downside of this life-giving hormone is its role in female cancers, which result from unrestrained cell growth in the breasts, uterus, or ovaries. Even before matters get to this stage, however, excess estrogen can create deficiencies of zinc, magnesium, and B vitamins. And when estrogen is out of balance with its partner, the hormone progesterone, estrogen dominance can result.

Even women with low levels of estrogen can suffer from this syndrome if their progesterone levels are correspondingly low. Men, too, can suffer from estrogen dominance, which, besides contributing to hair loss, fatigue, lack of sexual potency, and other signs of aging, may also put them at risk for prostate cancer. For both sexes, the symptoms of estrogen dominance can include the following:

Discomfort and Premature Aging

Allergy symptoms, including asthma, hives, rashes, and sinus congestion

Bone loss, even before menopause

Breast tenderness

Cold hands and feet caused by thyroid dysfunction

Decreased sex drive

Dry eyes

Fatigue

Hair loss

Headache

Hypoglycemia

Infertility

Irregular menstrual periods

Osteoporosis

PMS

Mental and Emotional Difficulties

Depression accompanied by anxiety or agitation

Foggy thinking

Irritability

Insomnia

Memory loss

Mood swings

Disorders

Autoimmune disorders, including lupus

Cervical dysplasia (a distortion of cervical cells that may be an early indicator of cervical cancer)

Fibrocystic breasts

Gallbladder problems

Increased blood clotting with an increased risk of stroke

Polycystic ovaries (another cancer risk factor)

Prostate cancer

Thyroid dysfunction, mimicking hypothyroidism

Uterine cancer

Uterine fibroids

And, if you're still wondering why it's been so hard for you to lose weight, you should know that estrogen dominance can also result in fat gain, especially around the abdomen, hips, and thighs; water retention and bloating; a sluggish metabolism; and a host of nutritional imbalances, including excess copper (the subject of my book *Why Am I Always So Tired?*), insufficient magnesium (a risk factor for heart attack, inefficient use of calcium, and bone loss), and deficiencies in zinc (related to the problem of excess copper).[13]

My own sense is that virtually all of us are suffering from estrogen dominance thanks to all the synthetic estrogens in the environment, as well as to the toxins that act like estrogens. Every time you're exposed to plastic, industrial waste, meat, soap, pesticide-laden fruits and vegetables, car exhaust, and much of the furniture, paneling, and carpeting in your home and office, you're setting yourself up for estrogen dominance.[14] As if that weren't enough, here are a few other sources:

- **Stress** increases the level of the stress hormone cortisol, which contributes to estrogen dominance. Cortisol also causes us to retain tummy fat, making it that much harder to lose both pounds and inches. Too much stress can interfere with our menstrual cycles as well, dumping excess estrogen into our bloodstream.

- **Medications** such as birth-control pills and hormone replacement therapy (HRT) deliberately add estrogen to our systems—for worthy medical ends, perhaps, but with troubling results for our weight and health.

- **Household chemicals,** including scouring powder, dishwashing detergent, laundry soap, fabric softeners, and window cleaners, contain numerous xenoestrogenic chemicals as do the pesticides you may be using in your home and garden.

- **Cosmetics and beauty products,** including shampoo, makeup, hair dye, hair sprays, lipstick, and fingernail polish and polish remover, may also include additives and preservatives that behave in a xenoestrogenic fashion and work their way into your system through your skin.

- **Environmental sources** of estrogen include not only the pollutants described above but also the estrogen-laden feeds given to cows and steers to help them—you guessed it—gain weight.

- **Water** in virtually every town and city in the United States is chlorinated, and chlorine is a major xenoestrogen. Whether you drink tap water or simply bathe, shower, or swim in it, you're exposing yourself to a fattening (and possibly carcinogenic) chemical.

- **Diet** is a big part of the excess estrogen problem for most of us Americans. A shortage of the phytoestrogens naturally found in plants like fruits (oranges, strawberries), vegetables (asparagus, Brussels sprouts, cabbage, radishes), seeds (flaxseeds), and spices (cinnamon, nutmeg, ginger) gets our system out of whack. When our bodies are supplied with enough natural plant estrogens, they more easily slough off excess estrogen into the bloodstream, which carries it off to be excreted in the urine. Ironically, insufficient estrogen from natural sources can cause our systems to become overloaded with estrogens from animal fats and artificial sources.[15] That's another reason why the Fast Track includes lots of fresh fruits and vegetables and healthy herbs and spices.

The diet–estrogen dominance link is even more pervasive. When we take in too many calories, we tend toward estrogen dominance,[16] and because the liver metabolizes estrogen, an overworked liver can also be dangerous to our hormonal health. We'll learn more about how the liver balances our estrogen levels in chapter 4. For now, let's just note that this is yet another way in which a detoxified liver is crucial to combating the xenoestrogens in our environment and to helping us control our weight.

I was one of the first to write about the problems of xenoestrogens and estrogen dominance in my book *The Living Beauty Detox Program,* a theme that was later taken up by bioenvironmentalist D. Lindsey Berkson, who conducted her own research about how the more than 3,000 chemicals deliberately added to our food can disrupt our hormonal balance and sabotage our diets.

In some cases, the synthetic chemicals Berkson describes seem deliberately intended to promote weight gain. She points out that in 1940, for example, farmers needed four months to grow a chicken; by 1990, they'd gotten the time frame down to six weeks. Although commercial farmers claim that genetic engineering is responsible, organic farmers need a full ten weeks to raise their poultry. That four-week difference may well be the result of artificial interference, which translates into our body's own extra pounds of chicken fat.[17]

Like Baillie-Hamilton, Berkson points out that estrogenic hormones are given to cattle to speed their weight gain. Moreover, she says, animal feeds are among the most heavily sprayed crops, loaded with pesticides, herbicides, and fungicides that, although they're not exactly xenoestrogens, can nevertheless disrupt our hormones and provoke weight gain. For an extra dose of bad news, she informs us that most animal feed contains rendered fat, which is often salvaged from fast-food restaurants. This melted fat tends to contain melted plastic as well, to further stress our livers and colons and disrupt our weight.[18]

Even the healthy fruits and veggies we consume may be setting us up for weight gain when they contain pesticides and other toxins. Berkson cites a study by the Environmental Working Group—the same organization that conducted Rome's body burden project—on the prevalence of these common poisons: "You eat small amounts of numerous pesticides, you quite likely eat them every day, and quite possibly in every meal." Recall, too, that such insecticides as DDT, banned in the United States, return to our bodies via foods imported from India, where DDT use doubles every eleven years, and Mexico, a heavy user of the product. The same report found that endosulfan had been used illegally on at least ten U.S. crops. It is significant, according to Berkson, that endosulfan mimics the behavior of estrogen in the human body.[19]

Many other environmentalists have warned against the effect of toxins on our hormones. A team of European toxicologists, for example, claims that "new chemicals with endocrine disrupting potential continue to be discovered, inadvertent forms of exposure are constantly being identified, and there is increasing concern about cumulative effects."[20]

Reversing the Trend

When I shared the information about chemicals and body weight with my group at the Learning Annex and then told them about the toxic effects of our environment, I could sense a chill coming over the room. Most of us may have some general sense that our planet is becoming more polluted, but few of us live daily with a vivid picture of just how many poisons are entering our bodies. And even fewer of us understand the problems that pollution causes for our weight as well as our health.

The good news, I told them, is that once we understand the problem, we can work to solve it. The first step is a good, healthy detoxification—a brand of detox that supports our liver and our colon while ridding our bodies of the toxins, xenoestrogens, and additives that we've accumulated. For years, in *Beyond Pritikin* and the *Fat Flush* series, I advocated detox through careful dietary choices—an approach I still recommend because *purifying diets help you lose weight.* And now there's a new weapon for your detox diet arsenal: fasting.

The One-Day Detox Diet is specifically designed to help rid you of the toxins you've been storing over the years. And it's also intended to build up your major detox organs, the liver and colon, so that they continue to filter out and eliminate the poisons, thereby allowing you to absorb the nutrients you need. After you've worked your way through the Seven-Day Prequel, the One-Day Detox Diet, and the Three-Day Sequel, you may even be ready to take it to the next level, making the kinds of lifelong healthy choices described in chapter 9. I hope your personal experience with detox will raise your awareness of the kinds of health and environmental problems we are creating for ourselves and future generations. The first step, though, is to give the Fast Track a try. You are likely to be in particular need of this detox program if you've been on a low-carb diet. How low-carb diets are polluting our bodies and sabotaging our long-term weight loss is the subject of the next chapter.

> *I couldn't believe just how easy this was. And I wasn't hungry! I feel great! As a mother of five, I really appreciate that my energy was great, and so was my mental clarity. This was a perfect jump-start to starting a long-term eating plan.*
> —RENEE CERIO, THIRTY-SEVEN; LOST 2.5 POUNDS

3

Low-Carb Diets:
Making the Problem Worse

Awareness is curative.
—Fritz Perls

My client Mercedes was concerned. She'd come to me because she'd started experiencing a host of disturbing symptoms: acne, hemorrhoids, rectal itching, gas, bloating, and constipation. Her skin tone wasn't good, and she didn't have the energy she was used to. Her fingernails were starting to peel, chip, and break more frequently, and she'd noticed that more hair than usual was coming out in the shower. Plus she felt tired, dragged out, and cranky.

When I asked Mercedes about her eating habits, she explained that she'd been on a very low-carb, high-protein diet for about six months. That was another source of frustration, she told me: When it came time to start adding some carbohydrates back into her diet, her weight had immediately begun to creep up.

I told Mercedes that many of her symptoms were, in my view, signs of toxicity—the inevitable result of the twentieth-century environmental assaults you've just read about in chapter 2. Just think, I told her, industry introduces more than a thousand brand-new chemicals into the atmosphere each year—that's something like three new chemicals a day.

To make matters worse, these pesticides and new chemicals are not just your run-of-the-mill pollutants. They are that special breed known as xenoestrogens, which duplicate some of the effects of estrogen, the female hormone. They work their way into our food, cosmetics, homes, and workplaces, where they disrupt our hormones and increase our weight, besides producing the ugly and unpleasant symptoms she had just described.[1]

Mercedes's problem was further compounded by her high-protein, low-carb diet, which had loaded her up with the most toxic food source of all—hormone- and pesticide-laden animal proteins. At the same time, her regime had deprived her of the fruits, vegetables, and whole grains whose fiber, vitamins, minerals, and antioxidants she desperately needed to fight those toxins. To restore both her health and her ability to lose weight, Mercedes would have to detoxify, supporting her liver and colon so that they could expel the poisons from her system.

Mercedes agreed to try the Fast Track One-Day Detox Diet, fortifying her liver, unclogging her stagnant colon, and starting to clear her body of the poisons she had accumulated. When I saw her two weeks later, the difference was apparent. Her skin had started to clear, her hair had already begun to feel thicker, and her nails had grown in strong and hard. She'd lost 4 pounds on the Fast Track, and she was optimistic about continuing to lose weight with this new approach to eating. Best of all, she told me, she'd regained her normal energy levels, and maybe even a little bit more.

"I don't think I realized how much all that protein on my low-carb diet was weighing me down," she said. "Even though I was losing weight, I *felt* heavy, somehow. Now, I feel clean."

Toxic Invaders: How Low-Carb Dieting Puts Us at Risk

It's a well-known fact: The highest concentration of pesticides and other toxins in our diet comes from meat and dairy products. That's because animals store toxins the same place we do—in their fat. When we eat these polluted animals and their by-products, we are consuming the poisons that they were exposed to, in their feed, in their grazing area, and in their toxin-laden farm environment.

Now, I would never counsel you to give up meat, cheese, or eggs. On the contrary, high-quality sources of these animal proteins are a mainstay of the Fast Track, as you will see in chapter 5. But low-carb diets go to the other extreme. Their overemphasis on animal proteins, and their complete lack of consciousness about the need to choose organic meats, "clean" fish, and hormone-free dairy, puts you at increased risk from the toxic invaders you read about in chapter 2.

As we saw in that chapter, conventional animal feeds are among the crops sprayed most heavily with pesticides, herbicides, and fungicides. These agricultural chemicals have potentially toxic effects as well as tending to disrupt our hormones and interfere with weight loss. Thus up to 95 percent of all pesticide residues are found in meat and dairy products, according to the EPA.[2] So eating lots of meat, eggs, and dairy products—especially if you're not choosing organic foods—hugely increases your exposure to toxins.

Moreover, low-carb diets are sadly lacking in phytonutrients, crucial food elements found only in fresh fruits and vegetables.[3] Plant foods are rich in antioxidants—vitamins, minerals, and other nutritional elements that fight *oxidative stress*, in which cells are destroyed, the immune system is weakened, inflammation occurs, and aging accelerates. As we'll see in chapter 4, your liver needs big-time antioxidant support to sustain the body's major detoxification pathways. If you're focusing on pesticide- and hormone-laden meats while avoiding cleansing fruits and veggies, you're setting yourself up for a toxic invasion.

Low-carb plans that steer dieters away from fruits and veggies likewise lack potassium, that mineral so essential to keeping our blood pressure low and our heart beating regularly. Potassium also supports our adrenal glands and our nervous system, making it a basic mineral for supporting our energy and our mood.

Perhaps most important, however, we need the fiber found in fruits, vegetables, and whole grains to bind with toxins and expel them from our system.[4] A low-carb diet is by definition a low-fiber diet. Ironically, low-carb diets increase our exposure to environmental toxins by eliminating the body's best defense, all in the name of reducing carb grams.

If this is bad for our health, it's worse for our weight. A clogged colon can cost you several pounds as it loads up with impacted fecal matter. When you're not digesting food properly, you need to eat more to get the same nutrients and to feel "full."

These problems would be bad enough for people remaining at their current weight. But dieters who lose up to 20 pounds in the first five months on a low-carb diet have virtually doubled their exposure to toxic material. Not only are they eating animal fats that are high in toxins, but they are exposing themselves to these dangerous substances a second time when their own "animal fat" melts away. Moreover, if they're suffering from the constipation and impaired elimination so common on these low-fiber programs, they're attacked from a third quarter as well—the clogged, rotting fecal matter stuck within their own colons. The toxins are mounting, even as the fiber needed to help scrub those toxins away has been banned from their diets.

When I explained all of this to Mercedes, it was like a revelation. Her low-carb diet had put her at risk for symptoms that she'd never before experienced, so that even as she was losing weight she was also suffering from new problems. To add insult to injury, she had reached the point at which she had trouble losing weight or even maintaining the weight loss she'd already achieved.

Mercedes was luckier than she realized, though. There was one other common problem of low-carb diets that she had somehow managed to escape. My client Jewelle was not so lucky.

Low Stomach Acids: The X Factor in Low-Carb Diets

When Jewelle came to see me, she was nearly in tears.

"I don't understand why I'm having such a hard time digesting my food," she said. "I used to be able to eat anything, and now I'm just gassy and uncomfortable every time I finish a meal. Plus"—she lowered her voice as though she were admitting something shameful—"I have bad breath like you wouldn't believe. My boyfriend said something about it to me the other day, and I was so embarrassed! I don't understand why I'm having these problems."

As I questioned Jewelle further, I found out what I had already begun to suspect. Jewelle had started a low-carb diet a few months earlier, an Atkins-style approach that involved eating lots of protein and very few fruits and vegetables. For her, the change was particularly dramatic, because she had been, as she put it, "a real carb junkie" before she'd started the program. Suddenly, instead of relying on pasta, breads, and potatoes to fill her up, she'd switched to beef, chicken, and cheese.

At first, she said, it felt wonderful. The high protein content of her diet had given her lots of energy, and she'd dropped several pounds right away.

But then her troubles began. Gas, bloating, and the bad breath she was so embarrassed about had set in, as well as severe heartburn after almost every meal. Although she'd taken some antacid tablets for the heartburn, they seemed to make her feel even worse.

"No wonder," I told her. "Your problem isn't too much stomach acid, but too little. All that protein on the low-carb diet, plus the lack of fruits and veggies, means that you're putting a huge strain on your stomach acid production without giving your system the vitamins and minerals it needs to make more stomach acid. I don't think your high-carb diet was so healthy, either, but at least it didn't put this kind of strain on your stomach."

I suggested that Jewelle take some betaine hydrochloric acid (HCl) tablets supplemented with pepsin and bile extract to help restore her stomach acids. I also told her about the Fast Track. The Liver-Loving and Colon-Caring Foods in the Seven-Day Prequel would help provide the nutrients she was missing, I explained, while the One-Day Detox Diet would begin an internal cleansing process, helping get rid of the toxins lurking in her meat and cheese. I pointed out that betaine HCl, pepsin, and bile supplements are part of the Three-Day Sequel of my Fast Track, but that in her case, she might start taking them immediately.

Jewelle came to see me the week after she'd completed the Fast Track. She reported with relief that her symptoms had cleared up as soon as she'd begun taking the tablets. And the Seven-Day Prequel and Three-Day Sequel had given her a new appreciation of fruits and veggies.

"I feel like my entire body is breathing a huge sigh of relief," she told me. "I still want to lose weight—but not the low-carb way. It's just not worth it."

Are You Suffering from Insufficient Stomach Acid?

As Jewelle discovered, low-carb diets load dieters' systems with excessive amounts of protein that many people have difficulty digesting. As a result, they exhaust their store of stomach acid, and symptoms like Jewelle's are the results.

Diagnosing insufficient stomach acid is a tricky problem, because the symptoms for too little stomach acid are often the same as those for too much. So let's find out if you may be suffering from this oft-misunderstood problem. Take the following quiz to see how your stomach acid is holding up.

1. Do you have . . .

. . . food that seems to just sit in your stomach?

. . . the sense of feeling full after only a few bites?

. . . an unexplained loss of appetite, particularly the loss of a taste for meat?

. . . belching?

. . . bloating right after you eat?

. . . flatulence an hour after you eat?

. . . frequent gassiness?

. . . frequent nausea?

. . . frequent vomiting?

. . . a frequent burning sensation in your stomach, or heartburn?

. . . heartburn so severe that it wakes you from sleep?

. . . a chronically irritated throat?

. . . a chronically sore throat?

. . . laryngitis?

. . . hoarseness in the morning?

. . . difficulty swallowing?

. . . inflamed gums?

. . . a frequent sour taste in your mouth?

. . . bad breath?

. . . chronic *Candida* infections?

. . . chronic intestinal parasite infections?

. . . dilated blood vessels in your cheeks and nose that look red or rosy (rosacea)?

. . . rectal itching?

. . . weak, brittle nails?

. . . thinning hair?

2. Have you been diagnosed with . . .

. . . gastroesophageal reflux disorder (GERD), also known as acid reflux?

. . . protein, calcium, magnesium, and/or iron deficiencies?

. . . rheumatoid arthritis?

. . . hyperthyroidism or hypothyroidism?

. . . chronic autoimmune disorders?

. . . abnormal intestinal flora?

. . . chronic hives?

. . . osteoporosis?

. . . weak adrenal glands?

. . . lupus?

. . . vitiligo?

. . . rosacea?

. . . chronic hepatitis?

. . . gallbladder disease?

✳ **Any one of these symptoms or disorders can be linked to insufficient stomach acid and the inability to properly digest protein and acid-based minerals such as calcium, iron, and magnesium. Because insufficient HCl production can tax your liver and your colon, some of these symptoms may also be related to the ones we described in chapter 2. Consult your health-care provider or simply take the HCl Challenge (page 50) to find out if insufficient stomach acid is robbing you of your protein and minerals.**

Stomach Acidity: The Key to Digestion

Americans are experiencing a virtual epidemic of digestive problems. We used to believe that people over the age of forty routinely lost 50 percent of their ability to secrete stomach acids. But my own experience with thousands of clients has convinced me that these days, just about everybody is suffering from insufficient stomach acid. Worry, stress, and the pressures of our fast-paced life tend to decrease stomach acid—and who among us has escaped the consequences? So let's take a closer look at why stomach acid is so important—and how low-carb diets work to deplete it. When you first decide to eat your lunchtime salad, your brain sends out a signal, alerting your entire digestive system to start producing the fluids, acids, and enzymes that enable you

TAKE THE HCL CHALLENGE

If you think you might be suffering from insufficient stomach acids, and particularly if you've been on a low-carb, high-protein diet, there are two ways you can find out more. One is to ask your doctor to give you the Heidelberg test, in which you swallow a small plastic capsule containing electronic monitoring equipment. The capsule has the ability to measure the pH of your stomach, small intestine, and colon as it moves through your system transmitting a signal that your doctor can interpret.

A simpler, low-tech alternative is to take the HCl Challenge. Before the next meal you eat, take a hydrochloric acid supplement that contains at least 500 to 550 milligrams of betaine hydrochloride and about 150 milligrams of pepsin. (The brand I personally use and have been recommending to my clients and readers for years is the Uni Key HCL; call 800-888-4353 or see "Resources" on p. 215. This product also contains 65 mg of ox bile to aid in the digestion of fat.)

After you've taken your first HCl tablet, notice how you feel. If you're producing enough stomach acid, taking this supplement will cause you to feel a bit of pain or warmth in your stom-

to break down the food into its various components and absorb the nutrients you need.

Just thinking about food gets your system going. Smelling and seeing food is the second step. The sight of that crisp Romaine lettuce and the smell of that pungent garlic-lemon dressing literally make your mouth water—or, to put it scientifically, the prospect of food induces the production of saliva (what the kids call "spit").

Your saliva is a major part of the digestive process, as it contains amylase, an enzyme that breaks down starches. Saliva also contains an element known as epidermal growth factor, which stimulates the growth of liver cells. Saliva helps you chew and swallow your food,

ach. You can relax—your stomach acid is sufficient to digest the food you're eating.

If you don't notice any symptoms or any worsening of the symptoms you already have, increase your dose to two HCl tablets at the next meal. If you're still symptom free, or if the symptoms you've already experienced haven't gotten any worse, continue upping your dose, a tablet at a time. As soon as you feel a burning sensation or warmth, you know you've gone too far. Drop back to the previous dose, and continue taking the supplement as needed. However, don't take more than five tablets, and modify your dose if you're eating less than usual.

After four months, you might experiment with reducing your HCl dosage. If you get good results, continue to reduce your intake of HCl until you are no longer taking it. If your symptoms return, go back to your previous dosage.

WARNING: Individuals who are on antacid medications should check with their doctors before administering this self-help test. Also, note that HCl should not be taken with anti-inflammatory meds such as Indocin, Motrin, Butazolidin, or aspirin.

which passes from your mouth down into your esophagus, a long tube that leads into your stomach.

Meanwhile, thinking about eating has triggered the flow of hydrochloric acid in your stomach. By the time your food actually reaches the end of its esophageal journey, your stomach is full of HCl, ready to dissolve the food.

Hydrochloric acid is a remarkably powerful substance. Outside your body, it could literally burn a hole in the tablecloth or eat right through an iron nail. Within your stomach, HCl acts as a natural antibiotic, your first line of defense against toxic invaders. I don't want to alarm you, but if you had a microscope, you could see that even the healthiest lunchtime salad is simply crawling with bacteria. It's HCl that neutralizes those organisms, along with yeast and *Helicobacter pylori*, the bacteria associated with gastric ulcers.

Drinking too much water, particularly cold water, during a meal or within two hours after it, disrupts the function of stomach acid. So does eating under stress, or quickly, or without sufficiently chewing your food. And if you're under enough stress for a long enough time, your overall production of stomach acid will drop to a dangerously low level. Insufficient protein, a shortage of A and B vitamins, a lack of zinc, and not enough iodine or salt can also deplete your HCl levels.

Low-carb dieters don't have to worry about too little protein or salt, of course. Quite the opposite. By overloading their systems with protein, they've given their stomachs an impossible challenge. Few stomachs can keep up with the enormous amounts of protein that low-carb dieters take in—and undigested food, indigestion, and constipation are the results.

You also need HCl to absorb calcium, magnesium, and iron. All the calcium supplements in the world won't prevent osteoporosis if your stomach acid levels are too low. Likewise, no iron supplement you'll ever take will enrich your blood if you don't have enough stomach acid to absorb this vital nutrient.

Understanding Acid Reflux

Low stomach acid also leads to GERD, also known as acid reflux, a condition that is reaching epidemic proportions in the United States. When you're suffering from this problem, the contents of your stomach back up into your esophagus. Both undigested food and the stomach acid that is supposed to digest it rise up into a place where they're not supposed to be. Nausea, vomiting, and the burning sensation of heartburn—literally, acid rising into your esophagus—are among the most dramatic results. You might also experience bloating, gas, belching, rectal itches, fatigue, and all the other symptoms listed in the quiz you just took.

Because acid reflux is so often misdiagnosed, I urge you to look at that list of symptoms on pages 47–48 very carefully. If you suffer from more than two or three, or if you suffer from any of them frequently or severely, it is likely that you have some version of acid reflux.

Jonathan Wright, M.D., a nutritional pioneer whom I have followed for years and who is also an expert on hydrochloric acid, has found that some 90 percent of his patients who suffer from acid reflux have too little stomach acid.[5] So you do the math. If you're suffering from any of the common acid reflux symptoms listed earlier, you're probably producing too little stomach acid as well.

Stomach Acid and Weight Gain

The bad news doesn't end there. Low HCl levels are also associated with a spastic pylorus, the opening to the small intestine. Ideally, food should pass from your stomach into your small intestine, accompanied by a steady flow of bile—a vital substance secreted by the liver and stored in the gallbladder to metabolize fats and aid in the digestive process.

A spastic pylorus, however, keeps bile from entering the small intestine, so that it backs up into the liver and gallbladder. Meanwhile, the pancreas, which regulates the release of insulin, is also suffering from the lack of HCl and bile. Pancreatitis—inflammation of the pancreas—is one potential result. Diabetes is another. Poorly regulated blood sugar, with all the attendant problems for appetite and weight gain, is a third.

All these digestive problems take their toll on the colon, leading to constipation. The partially digested food sits in your colon far longer than it should. Remember, high-protein foods come from animals dosed with hormones and steroids and fed on pesticide-laden grains. So now you're exposed to all the toxins the food originally contained *plus* to the new poisons released as this food rots within your colon.

What can you do to repair the situation? Well, reducing the amount of stress in your life is one key defense. So is allowing yourself the time to eat slowly and with pleasure, chewing your food thoroughly and savoring every bite. Not drinking during meals can also help, as can taking HCl and pepsin supplements.

But an ounce of prevention is worth a pound of cure, as our grandmothers used to say. So one of the best ways you can fight the national epidemic of heartburn, indigestion, and acid reflux is to eat a balanced diet, avoiding the low-carb, high-protein mania that is sweeping the country. The Fast Track ensures that you get the nutrients you need. It also helps detoxify your liver, cleanse your bile, and ease the strain on your colon. As Mercedes discovered, this approach to weight loss just makes your whole system work better. I strongly urge you to give it a try.

Gluttons for Gluten

Although Jewelle suffered a great deal from her low levels of stomach acid, she, too, was luckier than she realized. She had at least escaped yet another little-known problem with low-carb diets—gluten sensitivity.

Gluten is the "gluey" protein that gives grains their texture. Primarily found in wheat, rye, barley, and possibly oats, it can also be found, as you might expect, in breads, pastas, cereals, crackers, cookies, and cakes made from wheat, rye, and barley. But gluten lurks in far more places in today's processed-food diet. Hidden gluten turns up in food starches, emulsifiers, condiments, gum, baking powder, dairy products, toothpaste, vitamins, medications, grain alcohols (rye, whisky, bourbon, scotch), seitan and other soy products, pickles, soups, meat products, and countless others.

Now, for some lucky people, gluten poses no particular problem. But most of us Americans have grown up eating lots of wheat- and grain-based products, and now we're paying for it. Gluten sensitivity is becoming increasingly prevalent, and all the more dangerous because it is so frequently misdiagnosed.

The most serious response to gluten—and the only one recognized by most conventional physicians—is celiac disease, an autoimmune reaction that attacks the lining of the small intestine and interferes with the body's ability to absorb nutrients. Symptoms of celiac disease include diarrhea, fatty stools, bloating, and in some cases, acute abdominal pain—often accompanied by weight loss.

Studies show that 1 out of every 111 healthy adults in the United States suffers from celiac disease, as well as 1 in every 167 children.[6] Moreover, 1 in every 12 first- and second-degree relatives of celiacs suffers from the disease, as well as 1 in every 30 adults with celiac symptoms.

The problem is even more severe among adults who have no symptoms: So-called silent celiac disease eats away at their intestines until they're finally diagnosed with anemia, osteoporosis, or another autoimmune condition.[7] These silent sufferers have no idea that gluten is at the root of their problem.

Besides celiac disease, gluten sensitivity expresses itself in a number of other conditions, including colitis, gastrointestinal complaints, nervous system disorders, dementia, frequent unexplained headaches, and canker sores. Gluten sensitivity is also expressed through the skin, in psoriasis, dermatitis, and various other skin diseases characterized by red bumps, blisters, itching, burning, and stinging. There is even some evidence to suggest that autism and schizophrenia may be related to gluten sensitivity.[8]

Any of us might develop gluten sensitivity, but low-carb dieters are at particular risk. Manufacturers have found that they can cut back on carb grams by simply using "low-carb" gluten rather than higher-carb wheat flour in their products. Walk down the aisle of any major supermarket, and you're likely to see dozens of low-carb snack foods, pizzas, breads, baking mixes, tortillas, packaged foods, and cereals. Now read the ingredients. You will undoubtedly find gluten at the top of every list. If a low-carb dieter has any sensitivity to gluten at all, these packaged low-carb foods are tailor made to set it off.

The irony is that low-carb eating plans were originally intended to free dieters from adverse reactions to carbohydrates. But by loading up convenience foods with gluten, the low-carb world is setting up dieters for a whole new host of symptoms.

Cranky, Forgetful, and Depressed: The Low-Carb State of Mind

When Mercedes switched from her low-carb regime to the Fast Track, she noticed an immediate boost in her mood. She felt calmer, less cranky, and more clearheaded and alert. I explained to her that the switch resulted from the increased levels of a highly important brain chemical, serotonin. Insufficient levels of this chemical are involved in depression, sleeplessness, migraine, PMS, and impulsive behavior—including binge eating. Nice, high levels of serotonin, by contrast, produce a state of comfort, calm, and alertness.

Our bodies make serotonin from the amino acid known as tryptophan, which is present in whole grains, legumes, root vegetables, eggs, turkey, and some dairy products. To manufacture this essential chemical, our brains also need plenty of fresh fruits and vegetables as well as the essential fatty acids found in nuts and seeds. Garlic is also helpful in serotonin production.

Mercedes realized instantly that her diet had been sadly lacking in some of the key nutritional elements needed to make serotonin. "That's why I felt so cranky and low energy while I was on that diet!" she exclaimed. "And why I feel so much better now."

Psychiatrists and mental health professionals with whom I have spoken are particularly concerned about the way that low-carb diets restrict their patients' serotonin levels. They are struck, as I am, about the relationship between serotonin and weight gain, as well as the link between low levels of serotonin and addictive, impulsive, and compulsive behavior. Low levels of serotonin make it much harder to "just say no," which could be a factor in binge eating. In addition, people whose serotonin levels are too low may find themselves ravenous for carbs and sweet foods in a misguided effort to medicate their nutritional imbalance.

The solution for such serotonin-starved dieters is not to eat the refined sugar and flour that they crave—that just produces a sugar high, followed by a sugar crash, as carb cravers know only too well. But it's also no solution for the serotonin-deficient to unduly restrict their carb intake on a low-carb program, which may be setting them up for serious nutritional deficiencies as well as mood disorders, migraines, and other hormonal problems.

Instead, serotonin-deficient dieters would do much better with the healthy carbs found in root vegetables, whole grains, and legumes along with their eggs, turkey, and a modified intake of dairy products. They also should make sure to get more fresh fruits, green leafy vegetables, and garlic—precisely the Liver-Loving, Colon-Caring Foods I recommend for the Fast Track.

Not So Sweet After All

There are two more problems with low-carb diets, and they both concern the artificial sweeteners so prevalent in the low-carb world. Both the sugar alcohols and sucralose (Splenda) are threatening low-carb dieters with a whole host of new concerns.

The sugar alcohols known as maltitol, xylitol, sorbitol, and mannitol are partially fermented substances that taste like sugar but are metabolized in a very different way, which leads to major gas, hours-long bloating, and even diarrhea in many people. Mannitol is the worst culprit—it sits in the gut longer than any other sugar alcohol. As a result, if you treat yourself to two or three low-carb candy bars, you will have easily consumed 20 grams or more of the stuff that can cause diarrhea.

The intestinal problems are bad enough. But there's also a potential weight issue. Sugar alcohols are generally listed on the package as having zero carb content. If your metabolism cooperates, this may be true. But if you happen to be one of those people who metabolize sugar alcohols differently, you may be getting more carbs than you realize. If you're an insulin-resistant or otherwise carb-sensitive individual—a description that fits some 90 million Americans or one third of the U.S. population—you'll find yourself piling on the pounds.

So if you're still counting carbs, you must read the labels on low-carb snacks that contain sugar alcohols very carefully. Divide the amount of sugar alcohol by 3 and add the result to your carb count. In other words, a "low-carb" or "no-carb" snack cake with 15 grams of sugar alcohol should really be counted as having 5 grams of carbs.[9]

But it's not just the sugar alcohols that may threaten your weight. Sucralose is the sweetener of choice in every low-carb recipe book on the market today. It's used in every low-carb product where sugar alcohols aren't. As sucralose is a chlorinated sugar derivative, I suspect that it is related to our friends the chlorinated pesticides, a major source of xenoestrogens. We used to think that sucralose passed through the system undigested, but now we know better. The latest estimates suggest that up to 40 percent of the stuff is absorbed and probably stored—just like its xenoestrogen relatives—in your body fat. So my advice is, Stay away from Splenda.

Other artificial sweeteners may also lead, ultimately, to weight gain. A provocative study by Professor Terry Davidson and Associate Professor Susan Swithers, psychologists working at the Ingestive Behavior Research Center at Purdue University, suggests that artificial sweeteners disrupt the body's natural ability to count calories.

In a study published in the July 2004 issue of the *International Journal of Obesity*, the researchers discovered that rats had a powerful response to sweetness. When they were given high-calorie sweet foods, they seemed able to regulate their intake, apparently because of some kind of internal calorie-counting mechanism that led them to read sweet foods as more caloric. But, the researchers found, when rats were given foods that had been artificially sweetened, the rodents quickly learned that the sweet taste was no cue to stop eating.

Then, ten days later, the rats used to eating artificially sweetened food were given a chance to eat a high-calorie chocolate-flavored snack. If you've ever overindulged in chocolate yourself, I bet you can guess what happened. The "artificially sweetened" rats, used to eating as much sweet stuff as they wanted, overate on the high-cal chocolate. The control group—rats used to only naturally sweetened foods—ate more moderately.

Likewise, the rats seemed to have an internal mechanism that led them to correlate viscosity—thickness—with calorie density. Rats given a kind of chocolate pudding seemed to gain less weight than those given a kind of chocolate milk, even though both substances had the same number of calories. Apparently, the thickness of the high-calorie food helped the first group of rats count calories. Again, if you've ever overdone it with sodas or other sweet drinks, you'll know just how those rats felt.

These results led the researchers to express concern over the number of Americans consuming sugar-free sweetened products, which rose from less than 70 million in 1987 to more than 160 million in 2000. Over the same period, the consumption of regular soft drinks rose by 15 gallons per capita.

"Increased consumption of artificial sweeteners and of high-calorie beverages is not the sole cause of obesity, but it may be a contributing factor," Swithers commented. "It could become more of a factor as more people turn to artificial sweeteners as a means of weight control and, at the same time, others consume more high-calorie beverages to satisfy their cravings."[10]

Setting Ourselves Up for Success

So what's the solution? How can we avoid the trap of obesity and weight gain on the one hand and the seductive but dangerous low-carb "success" on the other?

The answer is one I've been promoting for the past twenty-five years, throughout every one of my twenty-four books: a wholesome balanced diet especially high in Liver-Loving and Colon-Caring Foods, supplemented with essential fatty acids and well supplied with energizing protein. This is the eating plan that will help us feel full and well nourished, avoiding the digestive problems, gluten reactions, and weight-loss plateaus that are an all-too-frequent part of the low-carb diet craze.

But eating the right foods is not enough. We also have to rid our bodies of the toxins that accumulate from our food, water, and environment. This detox process is all the more crucial for those of us who are losing weight, because the most deadly toxins are stored right in our body fat. Melting that fat away dumps the toxins into our bloodstream, unless we flush them out.

That's why I have said our new slogan is No Diet Without Detox! And that's why I developed the Fast Track and its One-Day Detox Diet specifically to help cleanse the toxins from our system and to nourish the liver and the colon, our key detox organs. The Fast Track offers you one of your best chances ever for both "miracle" weight loss and long-term weight maintenance, an approach to food and nutrition that will sustain you the rest of your life. It's an unbeatable combination.

> *I had good mental clarity during the fast and plenty of energy. I slept great that night, too. I wasn't hungry and that really helped me detox.*
> —DONALD BAYLIES, FIFTY-EIGHT; LOST 4.25 POUNDS

Why You
Must Prepare
for Your Fast

In the middle of difficulty lies opportunity.
—ALBERT EINSTEIN

My client Marcy was confused. I had just suggested that she try the Fast Track, both as a way to jump-start the weight loss she was looking for and to help purge her system of the toxins and pollutants that I could see were weighing her down.

Marcy was a lovely woman in her mid-twenties whose skin still showed traces of the acne that had plagued her throughout her adolescence. Although she'd been an energetic teenager, she felt that she was wearing herself out as an adult, working long hours as an associate at her law firm all week and then sleeping ten or even twelve hours every Saturday and Sunday. Disciplined and committed, Marcy tried to watch what she ate and make time for a regular workout routine, but she was discouraged by the sense that she was fighting a losing battle with both her weight and her energy level. I sensed she was also troubled by how much of her life was dominated by work and how little time she had for herself and the people she loved.

The Fast Track One-Day Detox Diet, I suggested, could clear her skin, restore her vitality, and help her rebalance both her hunger and her priorities. Marcy liked the sound of all that, but she couldn't quite get behind the idea of a day without food.

"I always heard that fasting was absolutely the worst way to lose weight," she told me. "Maybe you lose a little weight on that one day—if you can make it through! But then your metabolism is so messed up that you just gain it all back right away, and have an even harder time taking it off."

Without proper nutritional support, that was true, I agreed. But that's the advantage of the Fast Track. You begin with a Seven-Day Prequel, fortifying your liver and stimulating your colon to eliminate waste properly by eating Liver-Loving and Colon-Caring Foods; drinking lots of pure water; and avoiding such Detox Detractors as alcohol, refined sugar, gluten, soy isolates, caffeine, the wrong kinds of fats, and mold. On your One-Day Detox Diet, you drink a delicious spiced juice made of cranberries and citrus, with ingredients carefully chosen to blunt your hunger, balance your blood sugar, rev up your metabolism, and nourish your organs. Then a Three-Day Sequel helps ease you back into eating and ensures you get the fiber and water you need to rid your system of any remaining toxins. You seal in the results of your fast by consuming natural food sources of probiotics, which help restore the friendly bacteria you need to keep your digestive and immune systems working at optimum levels.

Marcy seemed skeptical until I told her that I myself have been using the Fast Track One-Day Detox Diet for the past year and a half—but only as part of an eating plan that includes a daily dose of Liver-Loving and Colon-Caring Foods. In fact, I explained, I use the One-Day Detox Diet periodically to rid myself of the "travel bloat" and toxic feeling I get from being on airplanes all the time.

"Think of this One-Day Detox Diet as a purification for your body, mind, and spirit," I told her. "But you're absolutely right—you can't just stop eating. You have to follow the protocol."

Marcy still seemed uncertain about why, under some circumstances, a one-day fast could be a supremely healthy choice, while under other circumstances, it posed real dangers to your health, metabolism, and weight-loss goals. I explained that the secret lies in understanding how your liver and colon work, so you can give them proper support.

Love Your Liver

After more than two decades working as a nutritionist, I'll admit it: I am in awe of the liver. As far as I'm concerned, this amazing organ nestled away in the right side of the abdomen has more than earned its name, which derives from an Old English word for "life." The liver is your key to life, even possessing the unique ability to regenerate itself. Although your liver may need up to two years for this regeneration process, you can rebuild this vital organ with the right diet and detox plan. The Seven-Day Prequel will help regenerate your liver with Liver-Loving Foods that will keep it running smoothly and promote its detoxification. But first, let's get to know a little more about your body's hardest-working organ.

A Living Filter

Your liver is your largest internal organ, responsible for a number of processes that help keep your body in balance. It regulates your blood flow, supports your digestive system, and, if you're a woman, keeps your menstrual cycles running in peak condition.

One of your liver's most important functions, and the one most crucial to your weight loss, is breaking down everything that enters your body, from the healthiest bite of organic food to the poisonous pesticides that linger on your salad; from the purest filtered water to a glass of wine or a cup of coffee; from your daily vitamin and mineral supplements to the blood-pressure medication that your doctor has prescribed. It's your liver's job to distinguish between the nutrients you need to absorb and the toxins that must be filtered out of your bloodstream. By the way, medications, even if they're beneficial in other ways, are experienced as toxins by the liver, so if you're taking any kind of medication—prescription or otherwise—that's one more item that your liver has to filter out.

To do its formidable job, your liver engages in a number of detox processes, including a complicated two-phase procedure. In phase 1, your liver mobilizes up to a hundred enzymes that bind with toxins and begin to oxidize them. Some of those toxins are neutralized or changed to a less toxic form. They go on to be eliminated from the body in various ways, and no harm done.

Other toxins, however, are changed into a *more* toxic form. These so-called intermediate toxic compounds have to be broken down further in phase 2, during which the liver transforms them yet again and binds them to an amino acid or nutrient. This is how your liver detoxifies heavy metals, many solvents, petroleum products, alcohol, and medications (including acetaminophen and penicillin), as well as some substances that the body makes itself, such as hormones.

There are two hazards to this two-phase process. One is that the toxic intermediates create free radicals—molecules that are missing one or more electrons. These incomplete molecules exert a powerful pull on electrons in other cells, creating the kind of cell damage that can lead to cancer, degenerative diseases, and aging.

Ironically, the harder your liver is working to detoxify your body, the more endangered your liver and other organs become, threatened by the influx of free radicals that result from liver detox. Because antioxidants are your best safeguard against free-radical damage, you need a healthy supply of the antioxidants found in colorful fruits, vegetables, herbs, and spices to support your liver during this process. For phase 1, you need zinc, along with vitamins A, B_1, B_2, C, and E. For phase 2, you need folic acid, vitamin E, selenium, manganese, and glutathione as well as the amino acids methionine, cysteine, glycine, glutamine, and taurine.

But there's a second danger to this two-stage process. The intermediate toxic compounds are often more toxic than the substances from which they originally came. So if your liver doesn't finish phase 2 detoxification of these intermediate compounds, your efforts at detox have just had the opposite effect: overloading your system with extra toxins.

All too often, your liver *doesn't* finish phase 2, because highly refined carbs (like white flour, white sugar, colas, and candies), nitrates, hormones, and preservatives interrupt the detox process. Another set of disruptors is the xenoestrogens you read about in chapter 2. And you'll get major disruption from liver stressors like caffeine, alcohol, smog, secondhand smoke, medications, hormone supplements (including the Pill and HRT), and an excessive use of antibiotics. Any of these elements can interrupt the two-phase detox process, causing toxins to build up in your system.

That's why, if you're asking your liver to do extra work, such as during the One-Day Detox Diet, it's *crucial* to give your liver heavy-duty nutritional support, supplying it with the Liver-Loving Foods it needs while protecting it from Detox Detractors. Otherwise, you could end your detox with a weaker system and an even more toxic liver than when you began. And because a poorly functioning liver contributes to weight gain and weight retention, an improperly done fast will leave you in worse shape than you were in before.

THE GRAPEFRUIT CONNECTION

Although orange juice and lemon juice support your liver's two-phase detox, grapefruit juice actually interferes with the process. That's why doctors often tell patients on blood-pressure medication, antidepressants, and other regularly taken meds to avoid grapefruit juice. Their livers need all the help they can get coping with the medications, which—although good for their health in other ways—put an extra strain on their livers' two-phase detox process. That's also why I'm suggesting you avoid grapefruit and grapefruit juice during the entire time you are on the Fast Track—from the Seven-Day Prequel to the One-Day Detox Diet through the Three-Day Sequel. Of course, anyone who's not on medication can feel perfectly safe consuming this delicious fruit at any other time.

Beautiful Bile

The liver, in its infinite wisdom, also produces bile, a crucial substance for the detox process. One of bile's main duties is to help our bodies break down the fats we need as well as to assimilate fat-soluble vitamins. Without bile, we couldn't convert beta-carotene into vitamin

A, nor could we make use of calcium. Bile lubricates our intestines and works with fiber to prevent constipation. Bile is also where the liver dumps all the drugs, heavy metals, xenoestrogens, excess sex hormones from the Pill and HRT, medications, pesticides, industrial chemicals, and other toxins so they can eventually be eliminated from the body.

The first problem arises when our bile becomes so congested with all these filtered-out elements that it can't function properly. It becomes thick, viscous, and highly inefficient in breaking down fat. As a result, you gain weight.

Meanwhile, if your liver isn't getting the nourishment it needs, it will have trouble producing bile in the first place. In that case, you'll have difficulty digesting and assimilating food as well as metabolizing fat. You may even develop an instinctive dislike for fats. I don't want to get *too* graphic, but if you're wondering about your bile levels, I suggest you check the color of your stool. A walnut brown stool means you're enjoying good-quality bile, whereas a light-colored stool lets you know your bile levels are low.

These low bile levels may also be the result of too many toxins. Remember that thick, viscous toxic bile? Well, when bile gets *too* thick, it has trouble moving through the bile ducts. It gets backed up in there, and you end up short on bile. Again, your fat isn't properly metabolized and, once again, you gain weight.

By the way, the liver makes its bile from bilirubin, lecithin, vitamins, minerals, fatty acids, and cholesterol. That's why you need *some* cholesterol in your diet. So when you're choosing protein sources, don't forget the eggs!

You can build up bile and support your liver by eating Liver-Loving Foods. You can decongest or thin your toxic bile by avoiding the Detox Detractors described in the Seven-Day Prequel. You'll notice the results immediately: better digestion, easier elimination, and a general sense of well-being. Improving your bile level will also help with weight loss, as you improve your fat metabolism, cleanse your system of excess fecal matter, get maximum benefit from the foods you eat, and feel fuller and more satisfied much earlier.

THE ESTROGEN CONNECTION

Remember the estrogen dominance you read about in chapter 2? As we saw, this newly burgeoning condition results from an excess of estrogen in the body, particularly in relationship to the hormone progesterone. Both men and women can suffer from estrogen dominance, but because women have such high estrogen levels, they are particularly prone to this condition— one symptom of which is weight gain.

If everything is working right, our bodies are continually making estrogens from cholesterol, our body fat, and some other substances circulating through our bloodstream. Ideally, the body's supply of estrogen is continually replenished, with new estrogens entering the bloodstream even as old estrogens are removed by the liver, put through the detox process, and eventually excreted through our urine and feces.

However, when your liver is toxic or even just on overload, it becomes less efficient about removing the old estrogens. In such cases, the old estrogens stay in our bloodstream while the new ones are added—and estrogen dominance is a result. As we saw in chapter 2, most of us are already on estrogen overload because of all the xenoestrogens in our food, cosmetics, homes, and workplaces. Our livers need to be able to cope with this excess burden; but if they're stressed, toxic, or missing key nutrients that support the detox pathways, they simply can't.

So that's another way in which an overworked liver is tied into weight gain and another potential weight-loss benefit from cleansing and supporting your liver. And it's yet another reason why you *must* eat sufficient Liver-Loving Foods during the Seven-Day Prequel while avoiding the Detox Detractors.

Caring for Your Colon

Your liver is your major detox organ. Like the oil filter for a car, it tries to remove the gunk and sludge from your system. Your colon, on the other hand, is your body's plumbing system. A high-functioning colon will efficiently expel waste from your body, keeping you healthy, symptom free, and ready to lose weight. But if your colon is clogged and toxic, as so many of our colons are, you're likely to encounter health problems as well as weight issues.

Ideally, food should remain in your system for only twelve to eighteen hours before your colon eliminates it as waste. Most U.S. adults, however, retain waste for two to seven days—with disastrous results for their health. The longer those waste products sit in your colon, the more opportunity for toxins to penetrate back into your bloodstream, where your poor, overworked liver has to deal with them all over again. As a result, your body, especially your fat, becomes overloaded with toxic residues.[1]

Unfortunately, the wrong kind of diet makes it more difficult for the colon to do its job. For example, your colon normally produces a certain amount of mucus to help move the feces along. But when toxins, drugs, medication, stress, or other factors irritate your colon, your organ protects itself by producing excess mucus. If you've been eating refined flour or sugar, its gluey, starchy residue binds with the excess mucus to create a layer of hardened feces that builds up on your colon walls. The delicate little villi—waving hair-like stalks that line your colon and are designed to absorb nutrients and transport them into the bloodstream—become encased in this fecal layer. And the more your colon becomes encrusted with impacted feces, the narrower the opening for your bowel movements. Between the hardened old feces and the slow-moving new waste material, you've created a toxic breeding ground for bacteria and parasites.

Constipation is one possible result. And clearly, constipation is a big problem in this country; we currently spend over $700 million annually on laxatives, and doctors log nearly 3 million visits each year from patients concerned about this issue. But even if you're regular, or suffer from diarrhea, you might still have a "dirty colon." And if you've been consuming lots of meat, chicken, and dairy products (as is recommended on an Atkins-type low-carb diet), your colon is soon buried under a load of putrefying protein.

Many conventional doctors deny that fecal matter accumulates in this way and downplay the dangers of a toxic colon. But I look at the rise of colon-related illnesses, including Crohn's disease, diverticulitis, colitis, and colon cancer, and draw what to me is an obvious conclusion: Our clogged, toxic colons are putting us at risk.

It's not just bodily wastes that are festering in your colon, either. Heavy metals, pollutants, and the remains of drugs and medication can stay behind with the other waste, releasing their toxins into the poisonous mixture.

You saw in chapter 2 the kinds of symptoms that might result from a clogged or toxic colon. Even if you are symptom free, however, a poorly functioning colon will weigh you down. You may literally be carrying extra pounds in excess fecal matter, which from the outside looks like tummy fat but which from the inside looks like fecal sludge or dried, encrusted fecal matter. Adding insult to injury, this encrustration keeps you from getting the most out of the food you eat, preventing your body from fully absorbing and assimilating nutrients. Many people notice that when their colons are cleansed, they can eat 1/3 to 1/2 the amount they were used to before, yet feel even more satisfied, energized, and nourished.

Fabulous Fiber

If toxicity is the problem, fiber is the solution. Fiber is the tough material that gives plants their structure—what our folks used to call "roughage." Fiber is nature's own detoxifier, literally scrubbing the clogged fecal matter out of your colon and off your intestinal walls, helping you stay regular, and enabling your colon to work at peak efficiency.

Fiber comes in two forms. *Insoluble* fiber, as the name suggests, doesn't dissolve. Bran, cellulose, hemicellulose, lignans, and other substances in seeds, veggies, and whole grains pass through our digestive tracts intact, carrying toxins and fecal matter with them.

Soluble fiber has a viscous, gooey texture and will partially dissolve in water. This is the type of fiber that softens our feces so that they move more easily through our bowels. Soluble fiber also nourishes the friendly bacteria that our gut needs to maintain healthy digestion and immunity. Gum, pectin, and psyllium—found in apples, berries, legumes, oats, nuts, pears, and some seeds—are all sources of soluble fiber.

Fiber of both types slows down the rate at which we metabolize food—a crucial factor in balancing our blood sugar. Fiber also speeds our food's progress through the digestive tract, so that it doesn't sit in our stomachs, intestines, or colon, breeding toxins and creating the problems we've just discussed.

Unfortunately, most Americans are eating far too little fiber—an average of 12 grams a day, down from the 30 to 40 grams that our grandparents ate. Yet a high-fiber diet has been shown to help prevent heart disease, diabetes, diverticular disease, and obesity.

Because the colon is my favorite organ, I've always stressed the importance of fiber, which is a centerpiece of the Fast Track. I've understood for a long time that fiber speeds digestion and elimination, slows metabolism, and helps us feel fuller and more satisfied from the food we eat. Soluble fiber taken before meals in water or juice induces the fiber to bind to the water in the stomach and small intestine, forming a gluey mass that not only slows down the absorption of glucose (the natural sugars in food that affect our blood sugar) but also keeps calories from being absorbed. Soluble fiber also helps lower cholesterol levels.

I think of the toxic colon as being a garbage dump in your system after the sanitation crew has gone on strike. The garbage just keeps piling up. Fiber, on the other hand, is the garbage truck that finally carries away the rotting food and toxic waste, restoring your system to cleanliness and health.

THE MANY BENEFITS OF COLON DETOX

- Smoother and faster passage of waste products through the system
- More regular elimination, with less strain
- Reduction or elimination of putrefying matter within the colon, with a consequent drop in the toxins that recirculate throughout your system
- Cleaning away old fecal matter that is stuck to your colon walls or in pockets within your bowels
- Drawing out poisons, toxins, heavy metals, chemicals, and drug residue
- Healing the mucous membrane that lines your colon and digestive tract
- Promoting "friendly bacteria" and flora within the colon (for more on friendly bacteria, see chapter 8)
- destroying and eliminating parasites
- reducing *Candida* overgrowth[2]

Ready, Set, Glow!

Marcy appreciated the mini science lesson I gave her, and she was happy to learn more about how the Fast Track would support her liver and her colon while she fasted. She also realized—as I hope you will, too—how important it was to support her liver and her colon *all* the time, not only when she was preparing for a fast. Armed with the dietary suggestions (discussed in the next chapter), she was ready both for her One-Day Detox Diet and for the rest of her life.

I work in a grocery store and was able to not be tempted by all the food. I go to work at 5 A.M. At 9 A.M. I usually take a break and get something to eat. I started to get hungry then, but I kept drinking the cranberry water mixture and I got over that point of hunger. I noticed that my stomach went down in size, and I am not bloated. I like the thought of cleaning out my system. It sure worked for me—I lost pounds and could see it on my own scales.

—CINDY FICCARO, FORTY-SEVEN; LOST 4 POUNDS

Getting Ready:
The Seven-Day Prequel

*Before everything else,
getting ready is the secret of success.*
—HENRY FORD

THE FAST TRACK PREQUEL—SEVEN DAYS

Prepare for Your One-Day Detox Diet with This Simple Six-Step Program

I. EACH DAY, CHOOSE AT LEAST ONE LIVER-LOVING FOOD FROM EACH GROUP:

1. **The Crucifers (1/2 cup cooked or 1 cup raw, about the size of a small fist)**
   cabbage, cauliflower, Brussels sprouts, broccoli, broccoli sprouts

2. **Green Leafy Vegetables and Herbs (1/2 cup cooked or 1 cup raw)**
   parsley, kale, watercress, chard, cilantro, beet greens, collards, escarole, dandelion greens, mustard greens

3. **Citrus (1 orange or the juice of 1/2 a lemon or lime)**
   orange, lemon, lime

4. **Sulfur-Rich Foods**

   garlic (at least one clove, minced), onions (1/2 cup cooked), eggs (2), daikon radish (1/4 cup sliced, either raw or cooked)

5. **Liver Healers**

   artichoke (1 small artichoke or 4 cooked artichoke hearts), asparagus (1/2 cup cooked), beets (1/2 cup cooked or 1 cup raw), celery (2 medium stalks), dandelion root tea (1 to 2 cups), whey (1 to 2 scoops), nutritional yeast flakes (1 to 2 teaspoons)

II. EACH DAY, CHOOSE AT LEAST TWO OF THE FOLLOWING COLON-CARING FOODS:

powdered psyllium husks (1 to 2 teaspoons in 8 ounces of water), milled or ground flaxseeds (2 to 3 tablespoons), carrot (1 small raw), apple (1 small raw with skin), pear (1 small raw with skin), berries (1 cup)

III. EACH DAY, DRINK HALF YOUR BODY WEIGHT IN OUNCES OF FILTERED OR PURIFIED WATER.

IV. EACH DAY, MAKE SURE YOU HAVE AT LEAST TWO SERVINGS (THE SIZE OF THE PALM OF YOUR HAND) OF PROTEIN IN THE FORM OF LEAN BEEF, VEAL, LAMB, SKINLESS CHICKEN, TURKEY, OR FISH, OR, IF YOU'RE A VEGAN OR VEGETARIAN, AT LEAST 2 TABLESPOONS A DAY OF A HIGH-QUALITY BLUE-GREEN ALGAE OR SPIRULINA SOURCE.

V. EACH DAY, MAKE SURE YOU HAVE 1 TO 2 TABLESPOONS OF OIL IN THE FORM OF OLIVE OIL, FLAXSEED OIL, OR THE WOMAN'S OIL (A FLAXSEED OIL–BLACK CURRANT OIL BLEND).

VI. AVOID THE FOLLOWING DETOX DETRACTORS:

- *Excess fat,* especially trans fats from margarine and processed and fried foods

- *Sugar and all its relatives,* including high-fructose corn syrup, honey, molasses, maple syrup, sugar cane crystals, pure sugar cane juice, evaporated cane juice, dried cane juice, maltodextrin, and all products ending in "-ose" (such as sucrose, dextrose, fructose, and levulose)

- *Artificial sweeteners,* including aspartame, sucralose or Splenda, and sugar alcohols (such as maltitol, mannitol, sorbitol, and xylitol)

- *Refined carbohydrates,* including white rice and products made from white flour

- *Gluten,* found in wheat, rye, barley, and all their products (including breads, pastas, crackers, and crusts); also found in many "low-carb" products (such as packaged cereals, macaroni and cheese, pizza dough mix, spaghetti, shells, tortillas, pancake/waffle mixes, and cookies) and in vegetable proteins, modified food starch, some soy sauces, and distilled vinegars

- *Soy protein isolates,* found in low-carb "energy" bars and soy protein powders; and processed soy foods (such as soy milk, soy cheese, soy ice cream, soy hot dogs, and soy burgers)

- *Alcohol; over-the-counter drugs; and caffeine,* including coffee, tea, sodas, and chocolate

- *Mold,* found on overly ripe fruits (especially melons, bananas, and tropical fruits)

WARNING: If you do not follow the Prequel for the full seven days, please do not attempt the One-Day Detox Diet. You might end up more bloated, constipated, and "toxic" than you were before, which could put a halt to your weight-loss efforts. Fasting without prior liver and colon support releases into your bloodstream the toxins that were previously lodged in your fat cells. These poisons can then relocate and settle in any number of organs, making you feel tired, anxious, headachy, and more fatigued than when you started. You'll also be likely to gain more weight.

The Seven-Day Prequel: Preparing for Detox

Now that you understand why supporting your liver and colon is so important, let's take a closer look at how the foods in the Seven-Day Prequel are intended to do just that. To make it easier for you to get these Liver-Loving Foods and Colon-Caring Foods into your diet, we've got a whole chapter full of recipes (chapter 10) as well as an appendix devoted to resources (page 215) to help you find healthy sources of foods and supplements. We'll also include some tips along the way.

STOCKING THE STAPLES: YOUR SHOPPING LIST FOR THE FAST TRACK

- *Your choice of ten days' worth of crucifers:* cabbage, cauliflower, Brussels sprouts, broccoli, or broccoli sprouts

- *Your choice of ten days' worth of green leafy vegetables:* parsley, kale, watercress, chard, cilantro, collards, escarole, dandelion greens, mustard greens, or beet greens

- *Your choice of ten days' worth of citrus:* oranges, lemons, limes plus 2 oranges and 1 lemon to make the Miracle Juice

- *Your choice of ten days' worth of sulfur-rich foods:* garlic, onions, eggs, or daikon radish

- *Your choice of ten days' worth of liver healers:* artichokes or artichoke hearts, asparagus, beets, celery, dandelion root tea, whey, or nutritional yeast

- *Your choice of ten days' worth of Colon-Caring Foods:* powdered psyllium husks, milled or ground flaxseeds, carrots, apples, pears, or berries

- *Cranberry Juice:* 8 ounces of unsweetened cranberry juice or 1 jar unsweetened cranberry juice concentrate

I. Each day, choose at least one Liver-Loving Food from each group

1. The Crucifers (1/2 cup cooked or raw, the size of a small fist)
cabbage, cauliflower, Brussels sprouts, broccoli, broccoli sprouts

Cruciferous veggies stimulate the phase 1 and phase 2 liver detox pathways. Broccoli, Brussels sprouts, and cabbage enhance the process known as glutathione conjugation, in which the liver converts fat-soluble toxins into water-soluble substances that can be passed out through the urine.

Crucifers of all types also contain vital phytonutrients (nutrients

Recommended brands of unsweetened cranberry juice are Lakewood 100% Organic, Mountain Sun, Trader Joe's, and Knudsen. Recommended brands of unsweetened cranberry juice concentrate are Knudsen and Tree of Life. Be sure to look for juice that has no sugar, corn syrup, or other juices added, including apple or grape.

- *Spices:* fresh and nonirradiated cinnamon, ginger, and nutmeg

- *Stevia Plus*

- *3 days' worth of yogurt or raw sauerkraut or 1 head of cabbage, mustard seeds, cumin, and Morton's canning and pickling salt*

- *3 cups of fresh sprouts:* mung bean, alfalfa, radish, broccoli, or lentil (store-bought or homemade)

- *Optional:* the Fast Detox Diet Kit (see page 83) or individual supplements, including Liver-Lovin' Formula; Liver Care, or AFBeta Food; Super GI Cleanse; hydrochloric acid in a formula that contains at least 500 to 550 milligrams of betaine hydrochloride with about 150 milligrams of pepsin and 65 milligrams of ox bile; FloraKey or Dr. Ohhira's Probiotics 12 Plus

If you have trouble finding any of these products at your local supermarket or health-food store, see "Resources" (page 215) for information about where to buy them by phone or online.

found only in plants) such as indole-3-carbinol and sulforaphane, which aid the liver in neutralizing chemicals and drugs. For extra sulforaphane, try a few servings of broccoli spouts during your Seven-day Prequel. This little-known food is the highest known source of that miraculous compound, which scientists at Johns Hopkins University identified as supporting antioxidants and essential cellular function.

Remember how the two-phase liver detox process creates so many free radicals? That means antioxidants are a crucial form of liver support, and crucifers are an excellent source of the antioxidant vitamin C.

Tip: Broccoli sprouts can be purchased at fine health food stores under the brand name Brocco Sprouts. You can also find them online at www.broccosprouts.com. Pop them in salads, as I did in Layered Rainbow Salad with Broccoli Sprouts on page 189; use them on top of deviled eggs; or add them as a garnish for your steamed veggies.

2. Green Leafy Vegetables and Herbs (1/2 cup cooked or 1 cup raw)
parsley, kale, watercress, chard, cilantro, beet greens, collards, escarole, dandelion greens, mustard greens

Chlorophyll-rich greens are powerful blood purifiers and natural internal deodorizers. They're also a great source of magnesium, one of the minerals that helps the liver manufacture enzymes smoothly and efficiently. Your body also needs magnesium for over 350 cellular processes—and all of your 650 muscles need it every second of every day. Magnesium is an anti-anxiety mineral, a major muscle relaxant, and a natural laxative to boot.

The bitter taste of such greens as chard, kale, and escarole stimulates digestive secretions. In Asian medicine, bitter-tasting foods are considered to be particularly healthy for the liver, perhaps because of the association between bitterness and bile.

Cilantro is a savory herb known in alternative medicine circles for its mercury-chelating properties. New research now suggests that cilantro is also effective in eradicating *Salmonella*, the nasty bacteria that can cause illness and even death. (Pesto Presto Cilantro on page 190 is a zesty way to introduce your taste buds to this healing herb.)

3. Citrus (1 orange or juice of 1/2 fresh lemon or lime)
orange, lemon, lime

Oranges, lemons, and limes are full of vitamin C, perhaps the most liver-loving vitamin of them all. Vitamin C stimulates the production of glutathione, the liver's premiere antioxidant, which is crucial for a successful progression through the two-phase detox process. You can't take glutathione supplements by themselves because the molecules are too large to be absorbed by your gastrointestinal tract; so, if you want to be sure you've got enough of this vital antioxidant, load up on vitamin C. By stimulating glutathione, vitamin C also helps bind up heavy metals like mercury and cadmium and eliminate them from your body.

Vitamin C is also essential for acetylation, the process whereby the body eliminates potentially toxic sulfa drugs.

Tip: Squeeze lemon or lime juice into your daily dose of water, and try fresh lemon or lime juice to add some zing to your salads.

4. Sulfur-Rich Foods
garlic (at least one clove, minced, preferably raw), onions (1/2 cup cooked), eggs (2), daikon radish (1/4 cup sliced, either raw or cooked)

One of the processes by which the liver eliminates toxins is known as *sulfation*—so called because sulfur is an indispensable part of the procedure. These sulfur-rich foods make toxins easier to eliminate.

Daikon radish goes a step further—it also aids in the digestion and metabolism of fats. That's why in Asian cuisine, you're always served a bit of daikon with any fatty or hard-to-digest food. This long white radish, with its crisp texture and somewhat pungent taste, also acts as a diuretic and decongestant. Do check out the recipe Delightful Daikon Radish (page 193).

Eggs are rich in the amino acids methionine, cysteine, glycine, glutamine, and taurine. As we've seen, your liver needs these acids (also found in whey) to successfully complete phase 2 of its detox process. And eggs offer the lechithin your liver needs to produce that beautiful bile.

5. Liver Healers

artichoke (1 small or 4 cooked hearts), asparagus (1/2 cup cooked), beets (1/2 cup cooked or 1 cup raw), celery (2 medium stalks), dandelion root tea (1 to 2 cups), whey (1 to 2 scoops), nutritional yeast flakes (1 to 2 teaspoons)

Artichokes, especially the hearts, contain powerful antioxidants known as flavonoids that protect the liver's cells and tissues. Artichokes are also good for the secretion of bile, which, as we've seen, helps the body better digest and assimilate fats. The artichoke is a close relative of milk thistle, queen of the liver protectors, which offers major defense against free radicals and is especially good for people with compromised immunity or alcohol-related liver problems. If you're looking for more artichoke in your diet, you'll love Absolutely Artichoke Soup (page 194).

Asparagus contains high amounts of vitamin A and potassium, another mineral on which the liver depends during detox.

Beets are full of betaine, which helps protect the liver against the damaging effects of alcohol. Betaine also thins the bile and helps it move freely within the bile ducts.

Dandelion root stimulates liver function. It also contains inulin, a fiber-like substance that functions as a *prebiotic*—an element that helps nourish the friendly bacteria in the gut. As if that weren't enough, the humble dandelion root is also good for lowering blood sugar. I like the Alvita and Traditional Medicinals brands of tea.

Whey is a rich source of the amino acid L-cysteine, which, like vitamin C, is a precursor to glutathione. Little Miss Muffett may not have known how important whey was to keep her glutathione supplies high—but now *you* do. Remember, the liver's own two-phase detox process uses up huge amounts of glutathione, so it's up to us to replenish it daily. Whey also contains methionine, glycine, glutamine, and taurine—amino acids that are crucial to the liver's phase 2 detox process. I recommend Fat Flush Whey, made from milk that is hormone free.

Nutritional yeast is a complete protein that contains eighteen amino acids and fifteen minerals and is a stellar source of the B vitamins that are so necessary in both phases of liver detox. Vitamin B_1 helps decrease the effects of alcohol, smoking, and heavy metal toxicity. Vitamin B_2 is used in the production of glutathione. Vitamin B_3 is used in phase 1 detoxification. Vitamin B_5, also known as pantothenic acid, helps detoxify acetaldehyde produced from alcohol and by *Candida* overgrowth. This wonder yeast also includes vitamin B_{12}. Because vegetarians aren't getting this crucial element in meat, they need to make sure they get it another way—and yeast is a terrific alternative.

Nutritional yeast is not to be confused with the old-time brewer's yeast, a by-product of the process of making beer. Brewer's yeast is very bitter and contains wild yeast strains from the brewing process. It also tends to encourage *Candida* and yeast overgrowth. Nutritional yeast, by contrast, is a primary product grown on strains of mineral-rich molasses or cereal by-products. The best kind is grown on molasses or maple syrup, because the yeast absorbs the minerals from its host, making it perhaps the best natural food form of minerals available for humans. It's pasteurized to avoid the use of living yeast, so unlike brewer's yeast, it won't give you gas or lead to bloating. It also won't encourage *Candida* or other yeast-related problems.

I like the Kal and Lewis Labs brands, available in most health food stores.

Tips: You can use a tablespoon or two of the nutritional yeast flakes in tomato sauces and soups, dust it on popcorn, or stir a spoonful into sauces or gravies. When I'm feeling depleted, I like to take some nutritional yeast between meals for a quick get-up-and-go—a pick-me-up that's especially useful for people trying to stop drinking coffee or to avoid a sugar crash. The nutty flavor of the yeast flakes actually tastes pretty good when you mix a tablespoon or two into a glass of water; and I guarantee you'll get a boost of energy within ten minutes. Or take some nutritional yeast right before a meal to take the edge off of your appetite.

VARIETY IS THE SPICE OF LIFE

I wanted to keep this Seven-Day Prequel as simple as possible, so I've given you lots of leeway to choose the foods you like and find easy to prepare. But I also want to urge you to vary your food choices as much as you can. There's still a lot we don't yet know about nutrition, especially when it comes to the exciting new field of phytonutrients, which have remarkable healing benefits, warding off disease and promoting optimal health. The more different kinds of fruits and vegetables you eat, the greater your chance of getting the full benefit of all of Nature's phytonutrients. Still, if you find yourself eating the same green leafy vegetable seven days in a row, don't worry. The main thing is to eat one item from each Liver-Loving Food category. Enjoy!

II. Each day, choose at least two of the following Colon-Caring Foods

powdered psyllium husks (1 to 2 teaspoons in 8 ounces of water), milled or ground flaxseeds (2 to 3 tablespoons), carrot (1 small raw), apple (1 small raw with skin), pear (1 small raw with skin), berries (1 cup)

Flaxseeds are a two-for-one fiber source, because they contain both soluble and insoluble fiber as well as lignans—estrogen-modulating substances that have antiviral, antibacterial, and antifungal properties. Because of their effect on estrogen, flaxseeds are especially helpful for women suffering from PMS, perimenopause, and menopausal challenges.

I like FiProFlax, which is just flaxseeds, but I'm also quite fond of Men's FiProFlax, a combination of fiber sources made from cold-milled certified organic flaxseeds, pumpkin seed meal, and zinc sulfate. Produced by the company Health from the Sun, the organic flaxseeds it contains are further purified by an infrared lamp that kills mycotoxins (mold-containing elements) on the seed. See "Avoid the following Detox Detractors," page 87, for more on the dangers of mold. *Women take note:* Ignore the name and treat yourself to a zinc-rich source of fiber made from an organic source and already ground up for your convenience.

Tip: FiProFlax and Men's FiProFlax add a delicious, nutty taste when stirred into smoothies, yogurt, or cottage cheese and when sprinkled over salads.

Psyllium is a most reliable stool softener. It thickens rapidly when

THE FAST DETOX DIET KIT

Throughout this book, I've offered you're a range of options for everything you need to successfully complete the diet. But I also want to make it easy for you. So I've created the Fast Detox Diet Kit, which contains three main supplements you can use as your dietary insurance throughout the Seven-Day Prequel, the One-Day Detox Diet, and the Three-Day Sequel:

1. **Super-GI Cleanse: a source of colon-cleansing fiber plus herbs that target your eliminating organs**

2. **The Liver-Lovin' Formula: designed to support your liver**

3. **Flora-Key: a powdered source of probiotics for complete gastrointestinal health. (You'll read more about probiotics in chapter 8.)**

Although the Prequel, Diet, and Sequel last only eleven days, the Fast Detox Diet Kit contains enough ingredients to continue the cleansing and restorative process for up to a month. To order, call 800-888-4353, or see my Web site (www.fasttrack detox.com).

added to water, so drink it down quickly and follow it up with several more glasses of water. Make sure you're well hydrated if you're taking psyllium, as it can dehydrate the bowel.

The fruits and veggies I've recommended are not only a wonderful source of fiber but also a terrific way to up your vitamin C intake and your antioxidant quotient. You'll find these delicious foods filling, as well, a good way to put your hunger to rest while giving your taste buds a treat.

IF YOU DON'T NEED TO LOSE WEIGHT OR IF YOU ARE PRONE TO DEPRESSION (SEROTONIN DEFICIENT), YOU CAN ALSO CHOOSE FROM THESE SOURCES OF FIBER:

- *Nuts and seeds:* One serving would be a handful of almonds, walnuts, sesame seeds, pumpkin seeds, or sunflower seeds. Eat them raw or toast them yourself at home, but don't buy dry-roasted products, which are more likely to contain additives.

- *Friendly carbs:* A single serving is 1/2 cup of chickpeas, lentils, adzuki beans, pinto beans, or kidney beans or 1/2 cup of oatmeal or 1 small sweet potato.

III. EACH DAY, DRINK HALF YOUR BODY WEIGHT IN OUNCES OF FILTERED OR PURIFIED WATER

The many amazing health benefits from plain old H_2O are too numerous for me to go into here. I'll just restrict myself to explaining how water helps detoxify your system by carrying away waste products more efficiently and helping your liver, colon, and digestive system to do their jobs. Your blood is 83 percent water, and it needs a good volume of water to help it carry the toxins and waste products that we know travel through it and to transport the nutrients it carries to every part of our body. Our cells, too, need water to carry away their metabolic waste products. And of course, our colons need water to help with the crucial task of eliminating waste.

Throughout my years of nutritional counseling, I've been struck by how many of my clients have told me they've felt hungry when I could tell, from their symptoms and eating habits, that they were really thirsty. Try drinking a few glasses of water at least twenty minutes before a meal and see if you don't require less food to feel full. Notice, too, the refreshed, energized feeling that drinking lots of water will give you.

When you do drink, remember that water is best taken at room temperature between meals, though you can drink up to half a glass of water (4 ounces) during meals. Drinking too much of *any* liquid while eating can dilute your hydrochloric acid, which is so necessary in the digestion of protein and the assimilation of acid-based minerals such as calcium and iron. And wait until two hours after you've eaten to drink any more.

Most Americans tend to be dehydrated, drinking too little water and too much coffee, tea, and caffeinated soda. These all tend to dry us out, thanks to the diuretic properties of caffeine. If you wait to drink until you actually feel thirsty, you've waited too long: dehydration starts long before we're conscious of it. So make sure you drink at least half your body weight in ounces throughout your day. And don't substitute another fluid, particularly during the entire time you are on the Fast Track. It's *water* that your body needs. You may be surprised at how much better you feel when this need is finally met.

IV. EACH DAY, MAKE SURE YOU HAVE AT LEAST TWO
SERVINGS (THE SIZE OF THE PALM OF YOUR HAND)
OF PROTEIN IN THE FORM OF LEAN BEEF, VEAL, LAMB,
SKINLESS CHICKEN, TURKEY, OR FISH OR, IF YOU'RE
A VEGAN OR VEGETARIAN, AT LEAST 2 TABLESPOONS
A DAY OF A HIGH-QUALITY BLUE-GREEN ALGAE OR
SPIRULINA SOURCE

You already know you need protein for energy, muscle building, and many other vital functions—but did you know that protein is also

WATER, WATER, EVERYWHERE . . .

I wouldn't exactly tell you to avoid bottled water, if only because I want to make this Seven-Day Prequel as easy I can for you. But you should be aware that we have no quality-control standards in place for bottled water, which might as easily come from a polluted river as from a fresh mountain spring. So if you're really concerned about high-quality H_2O, your best bet is a home filtration system. I've found that the Doulton Ceramic Water Filter, a three-stage system, is the most effective water filtration device available. In the first stage, the tiny pores in the ceramic remove bacteria, parasites, rust, and dirt. The second-stage filter is made from high-density matrix carbon, which removes chlorine, pesticides, and other chemicals. In the third stage, a heavy metal–removing compound eliminates lead and copper. (For information on how to purchase a Doulton filter, see "Resources.")

There is one brand of bottled water I often take with me on the road: It's called HydroPro/Aqua Rush Water. This special drink is processed with patented technology that helps create optimum hydration. So for those times when you can't bring a thermos full of home-filtered water with you, try HydroPro/Aqua Rush Water.

crucial to the detox process? Protein activates the production of the enzymes that your detox system needs to break down toxins into water-soluble substances so they can be eliminated from the body. So when you're preparing for your Seven-Day Prequel, don't forget the protein! (*Vegans and vegetarians:* For more information on a top-notch brand of blue-green algae that I recommend, see chapter 9.)

I know many of you have been reading about safe vs. unsafe fish, and believe me, that's a concern I share. If you'd like to know more about which fish are safest for you to eat, look at the discussion of this topic in chapter 9.

V. Each day, make sure you have 1 to 2 tablespoons of oil in the form of olive oil, flaxseed oil, or The Woman's Oil (a flaxseed oil–black currant seed oil blend)

You need oil to lubricate your intestines, helping your colon more easily pass all waste products—and the toxins they carry—out of your body. Flaxseed oil and The Woman's Oil will also provide you with a healthy source of the fat-burning omega-3s, to aid in weight loss as well as detox. The Woman's Oil contains black currant seed oil, a source of the "good" omega-6s fatty acids, which is also a natural weight-loss aid and terrific for beautiful skin.

VI. Avoid the following Detox Detractors

- excess fat, especially trans fats from margarine and processed and fried foods

- sugar and all its relatives, including high-fructose corn syrup, honey, molasses, maple syrup, sugar cane crystals, pure sugar cane juice, evaporated cane juice, dried cane juice, maltodextrin, and all products ending in "-ose" (such as sucrose, dextrose, fructose, and levulose)

- artificial sweeteners, including aspartame, sucralose or Splenda, and sugar alcohols (such as maltitol, mannitol, sorbitol, and xylitol)

- refined carbohydrates, including white rice and products made from white flour

- gluten, found in wheat, rye, barley, and all their products (including breads, pastas, crackers, and crusts), also found in many "low-carb" products (such as packaged cereals, macaroni and cheese, pizza dough mix, spaghetti, shells, tortillas, pancake/waffle mixes, and cookies) and in vegetable proteins, modified food starch, some soy sauces, and distilled vinegars

- soy protein isolates, found in low-carb "energy" bars and soy protein powders, and processed soy foods (such as soy milk, soy cheese, soy ice cream, soy hot dogs, and soy burgers)

- alcohol; over-the-counter drugs; and caffeine, including coffee, tea, sodas, and chocolate

- mold, found on overly ripe fruits (especially melons, bananas, and tropical fruits)

These Detox Detractors either lower enzyme activity during phases 1 and 2 detox, interrupting the liver's efforts to transform toxins into nontoxic metabolites, or are linked to a decreased absorption of necessary detox nutrients. Therefore *you must avoid them* during the seven days before your fast, or you'll start your fast with an increased toxic load. Given this extra burden, your liver will be slowed down in its efforts to metabolize fat and detoxify your body, which will both impede your weight-loss efforts and leave you feeling sluggish, weak, and low energy. Here's a closer look at how each Detox Detractor works its evil magic.

Excess fat, especially trans fat, strains both your liver and your colon, so during the Seven-Day Prequel, avoid foods that are processed, refined, or fried, such as many cookies, candies, cakes, crackers, and crusts. You might even cut back on the "good fat" foods at this time—peanut butter and almond butter; excessive nuts, such as almonds, peanuts, and cashews; seeds; avocados; and even salad dressings, including the very best virgin olive oil, coconut oil, or macadamia nut oil. Any of these otherwise healthy fats can be hard for the liver to break down if your bile is congested or thickened with toxins. And, of course, trans fats are dangerous at all times, so stay away from processed vegetable oils, margarine, vegetable shortenings, and baked goods made from these oils. Happily, as of January 1, 2006, food labels will have to list trans fat content.

Sugar and other sweeteners, natural or artificial, stress both your liver and your colon. Moreover, both natural sugar and sugar alcohols have the potential to feed yeast, a known liver stressor because of the aldehydes that are formed—substances that overload the detox pathways and inhibit the action of the detox enzymes.

Refined carbohydrates, along with sugar, are deadly to both detox and weight loss. Not only do they inhibit the liver's detox pathways but they create those roller-coaster highs and lows in blood sugar, insulin, hunger, and cravings. Due to these blood sugar and insulin ups and downs the white stuff—whether sugar, flour, or white rice—is most likely to be stored as fat.

Gluten, as we've seen, is one of the big hidden dangers in low-carb diet products. As its name suggests, it creates a gluey substance that can bind with fat and mucus to cover the intestinal villi and clog your colon, which is particularly dangerous for those who have been on a low-fiber diet like Atkins (or like the typical U.S. diet). Gluten intolerance is more prevalent than previously recognized, so don't tempt trouble; during your Seven-Day Prequel, avoid low-carb products made with gluten as well as breads, wheat, and other gluten-bearing grains.

Soy protein isolates are incomplete proteins that lack the sulfur-bearing amino acids methionine and cysteine. The high-phytic acid in unfermented and processed soy products disrupts mineral absorption and can deplete your supply of zinc, magnesium, and calcium, which you need for liver detox. (Miso and tempeh, which are forms of fermented soy, are fine.)

Alcohol, drugs, and caffeine are liver stressors that tax the detox pathways big time. So definitely ax the alcohol, soft drinks, and colas—and avoid both regular and decaffeinated coffee as well as black and green tea.

Sadly, green tea is a no-no because an increasing body of studies has shown that it is contaminated with aluminum fluoride from pesticides and fertilizers. Fluoride cues your organs, including your liver and your brain, to stockpile aluminum, with sometimes disastrous results. Fluoride is also a known thyroid suppressor. With nearly 50 percent of the population suffering from hypothyroidism, and considering all the fluoride you're consuming in your water, toothpaste, soft drinks, and foods processed with fluoridated water, do you really want to take a chance on "fluoridated" green tea? Recent samples of green tea were also found to contain the pesticides DDT and its cousin, the DDT-like Dursban. Although DDT has been banned in the United States since 1972, it can still find its way back to this country from China or India in your teabag.[1] (If you really miss your tea, try a caffeine-free herbal blend, made from lemon, ginger, cinnamon, cloves, or cranberry. Teas like Celestial Seasoning's Bengal Spice, Cranberry Cove, and Lemon Lift are very satisfying choices.)

THE CAFFEINE CONNECTION

One of the hardest substances in the world to give up is caffeine, whether in the form of coffee, black or green tea, sodas, or chocolate. If you're used to a daily dose of caffeine, you may experience some withdrawal symptoms, such as headache, cravings, irritability, fatigue, depression, anxiety, nervousness, inability to concentrate, nausea, a runny nose, and sudden fluctuations in body temperature.

All the Liver-Loving fruits and veggies you're consuming will up the vitamin C in your diet, sustaining your adrenal glands—those major stress glands that bear the brunt of caffeine highs and lows. They'll also combat withdrawal symptoms to some extent. Meanwhile, drinking *half your body weight in ounces of water* will help you flush the caffeine from your system. You can also try taking The Adrenal Formula, a combination of glandular tissue extracts and nutrients that support the adrenals and contain tyrosine, which seems to be helpful in curbing detox withdrawal symptoms (see "Resources").

However you do it, I strongly urge you to kick the caffeine habit before your One-Day Detox Diet. Fast Trackers who gave up food *and* coffee at the same time ended up with caffeine headaches, mood crashes, mental fog, and fatigue on their fasting days. Ease your transition into a caffeine-free day by using this week to prepare.

Finally, avoid any unnecessary over-the-counter drugs at this time (but don't stop taking prescription meds without consulting with your doctor).

Mold can stress your liver, so avoid all sources of mold, especially moldy fruit, because some fruit molds produce mycotoxins that can cause severe liver damage, cancer, breathing problems, or allergic reactions. Since fresh fruit is more susceptible to mold, consider purchasing your fruit frozen. Remember to refrigerate cut fresh fruit within two hours after serving, and don't buy more fruit than you can use within a short time. Inspect your fruit closely for signs of molds or bruises, particularly melons, peaches, and nectarines, which are especially susceptible.

Cleansing for Body and Soul

Remember my client Marcy from the previous chapter? She had been a bit nervous about fasting, but she'd agreed to give it a try. Well, when Marcy returned to my office two weeks later, she looked like a different person. She was glowing, smiling, and 5 pounds lighter, and she'd also come to a powerful realization. Her One-Day Diet Detox had been a meditative experience, she told me, in which she'd realized that she was simply working too hard. She planned to talk to her boss about some simple ways to reorganize her work load that would enable her to keep up the office's demanding pace but still allow her some personal time. I was very pleased that for Marcy, the Fast Track had been both a physical and a spiritual renewal, a time for getting in touch with her true hungers—and her true satisfaction.

> *The juice really made me feel full. And my body feels much less sluggish now that I've done the fast. I know it was good for me to do it. It gave my body a chance to clean itself, and to create new cells. Best of all, I was not hungry! Thank you for this opportunity!*
>
> —MARILYN M. FINK, SIXTY-EIGHT; LOST 6 POUNDS

TOO BUSY FOR VEGGIES?
AN ALTERNATIVE SEVEN-DAY PREQUEL

It's always best to support your liver and colon with real, whole foods. But if you're on your own fast track and know you won't be able to follow the protocols in this chapter, there is an alternative. For your convenience, supplements are available; call 800-888-4353.

I. INSTEAD OF EATING LIVER-LOVING FOODS, TRY ONE OF THESE SUPPLEMENTS

- The Liver-Lovin' Formula contains a proprietary mixture of artichoke leaf powder (to support liver function), chlorophyll (to support purification), and L-taurine (a major amino acid detoxifier also necessary for the formation of one of the bile acids and for the proper breakdown of fats). Take 2 capsules, twice a day. (Note: This supplement is contained in the Fast Detox Diet Kit. See page 83.)

- LiverCare, the world's best-selling liver-support formula, was first introduced in 1955, with beneficial results reported in over 300 primary research studies. LiverCare has been clinically proven to be more effective than milk thistle in maintaining normal liver enzymes. I've found this product to be quite beneficial for more "heavy-duty" liver support, such as for people suffering from elevated liver enzymes, hepatitis C, fatty liver, and elevated bilirubin levels. Its main ingredients include caper, chicory, and black nightshade. Caper is a well-documented liver stimulant, whereas chicory increases bile secretion and promotes digestion. Black nightshade helps protect you against toxicity induced by drugs and chemicals. Take 2 capsules, twice a day.

- AF Betafood helps decongest both the gallbladder and the liver with its formula of dried beet juice. The betaine in the juice helps keep fats moving and supports their digestion, which in turn helps prevent their accumulation in the liver. Betaine also thins the bile and flushes out the routes along which bile travels, so that the increased bile drainage allows toxins to be eliminated more effectively. This wonderful product has been shown to help with bloating, gas, light-colored stools, hypoglycemia, diabetes, and elevated blood fats, as well as helping restore friendly flora (a form of bacteria) in the gut. People with severe liver problems—including elevated liver enzymes, hepatitis C, fatty liver, and elevated bilirubin levels—have also benefited from this product. Take 2 tablets three times a day, with or without meals.

II. Instead of Eating Colon-Caring Foods, Try This Supplement

• Super-GI Cleanse, which I helped formulate, contains five balanced sources of soluble and insoluble fiber from psyllium, flaxseeds, apple pectin, oat bran, and rice bran along with beneficial herbs, including butternut root, fennel, licorice, Irish moss, anise, and peppermint leaves. The herbs suppport the fiber by soothing digestion and helping eliminate wastes from all the body's elimination pathways—liver, kidneys, lymph nodes, and lungs. This product does not dehydrate the bowel as so many other fiber sources can. Take 3 capsules twice a day, upon arising and before bed, with 8 ounces of water. (Note: This supplement is contained in the Fast Detox Diet Kit. See page 83.)

III. Continue to Drink Half Your Body Weight in Ounces of Filtered Water

Whether you're eating natural foods or taking supplements, *you must continue to follow the water protocol.* You need that water to flush the toxins out of your system. If you think you're too busy to do even that, I urge you to slow down. All that rushing around is raising your cortisol levels, which is a major factor in retaining that tummy fat.

IV. Avoid the Detox Detractors

If you're used to depending on fast food, your morning cup of coffee, or a sweet bedtime treat, it's not easy to eliminate sugar, caffeine, and excess fats from your diet. But please give it a try. Consuming Detox Detractors the week before your One-Day Detox Diet is the best way to set yourself up for failure. Wouldn't you rather program yourself for success?

YOUR FAST TRACKER LOG: THE PREQUEL

DAY ONE

I. The Liver-Loving Foods I ate today

From Group 1: The Crucifers (¹/₂ cup cooked or 1 cup raw)
cabbage, cauliflower, Brussels sprouts, broccoli, broccoli sprouts

1. _____

Others: _____

From Group 2: Green Leafy Vegetables and Herbs (¹/₂ cup cooked or 1 cup raw)
parsley, kale, watercress, chard, cilantro beet greens, collards, escarole, dandelion or mustard greens

1. _____

Others: _____

From Group 3: Citrus (1 orange or $^1/_2$ juice of fresh lemon or lime) 1

orange, lemon, lime

1. _____

Others: _____

From Group 4: Sulfur-Rich Foods 1

garlic (at least 1 clove, minced), onions ($^1/_2$ cup cooked), eggs (2), daikon radish ($^1/_4$ cup sliced, either raw or cooked)

1. _____

Others: _____

From Group 5: Liver Healers 1

artichoke (1 small or 4 cooked hearts), asparagus ($^1/_2$ cup cooked), beets ($^1/_2$ cup cooked or 1 cup raw), celery (2 medium stalks), dandelion root tea (1 to 2 cups), whey (1 to 2 scoops), nutritional yeast flakes (1 to 2 teaspoons)

1. _____

Others: _____

II. The Colon-Caring Foods I ate today 2

powdered psyllium husks (1 to 2 teaspoons in 8 ounces of water), milled or ground flaxseeds (2 to 3 tablespoons), carrot (1 small raw), apple (1 small raw with skin), pear (1 small raw with skin), berries (1 cup)

1. _____

2. _____

Others: _____

III. The water I drank today

I need to drink ___9___ ounces of water.
Today I drank _____ ounces of water.

IV. The protein I ate today

1. _____

2. _____

Others: _____

_____

V. The oil I ate today

Today I consumed _____ tablespoons of healthy oil.

VI. Today I did/did not avoid all Detox Detractors.

My evaluation

How do I feel about how I stuck to the Fast Track today?

_____

_____

What strategies worked for me?

_____

_____

What will I do differently tomorrow?

_____

_____

Duplicate this log and use it for each day of your Seven-Day Prequel.

The One-Day Detox Diet

What would life be like if we had
no courage to attempt anything?
—Vincent van Gogh

WARNING:

Although fasting is an excellent link to better health for most
people, there are some times in your life when you should *not*
fast.

You should *not* fast if you are pregnant, nursing, recovering
from an illness or injury, debilitated, or malnourished, including those of you with AIDS, severe anemia, wasting states, or
cancer. People with weakened immunity should not fast.

You should *not* fast if you have cardiac arrhythmia, type 1
diabetes, congestive heart failure, ulcers, liver disease, or kidney disease or if you are struggling with mental illness (including anxiety, depression, bipolar disorder, or schizophrenia), as
your condition may worsen if you fast.

You should *not* fast before or after surgery, as it might com-
promise your ability to heal.

You should *not* fast if you are more than 10 pounds under-weight or if you are prone to an eating disorder.

You should *consult your physician and obtain permission to fast* if you are diabetic, hypoglycemic, or prone to severe migraines. Likewise *consult your physician* if you are taking regular medications, including antidepressants, blood-pressure medications, and birth-control pills.

Recently, I had the opportunity to talk with three dieters who were about to embark on the One-Day Detox Diet portion of the Fast Track.

Lucy was a marketing analyst in her mid-twenties. A warm, exuberant woman who had struggled with her weight since before she was a teenager, she told me that even the Seven-Day Prequel had been difficult for her to maintain. Her old pattern had been to use coffee as an appetite suppressant, drinking a few cups throughout the morning to enable her to skip breakfast and eat a light lunch. Then she would "reward" herself with a big dinner.

"I lost a couple of pounds just on the Seven-Day Prequel," she reported, "and although I'm still a bit groggy from giving up coffee, I did like eating all those fruits and vegetables. But a whole day without food? It makes me kind of nervous. I'm afraid I'll be hungry all the time."

Nila, a quiet, reserved woman in her mid-forties, had just returned to full-time work as a nurse after working part time and raising her children for the past ten years. "I often feel that I'm too busy to eat," she told me. "But my job is quite stressful, and on my days off, I have so many errands. I am concerned that if I eat nothing at all, I may simply collapse!"

Jason, a computer analyst in his early thirties, had been on my Fat Flush plan for nearly a year. He was pleased with how much weight he'd lost and how he'd been able to keep the weight off. Every so often, however, he'd indulge in a high-fat meal or a rich dessert, and given his sluggish metabolism, the pounds showed up immediately. For him, the One-Day Detox Diet was a kind of insurance policy, something he knew he could rely on if his weight began to creep up. Still, he admitted, he was used to a hearty breakfast, a good-size lunch, and frequent healthy snacks throughout the day. "I have this image of getting weaker and weaker, until by the end of the day, I'm just lying on the couch," he admitted. "I'd like to lose these extra pounds—and I'd *sure* like to know that I can always take off any extra weight. But how hard is it going to be?"

I was happy to reassure all three dieters that I'd specially designed the One-Day Detox Diet to address just these concerns. The Fast Track Miracle Juice, a delicious blend of cranberry and citrus juices spiced with cinnamon, ginger, and nutmeg, is composed of ingredients that would stave off hunger, balance blood sugar, and rev up metabolism.

I reminded these budding Fast Trackers of the experience of Anastasia Signoretta, the twenty-seven-year-old Fast Tracker whom you read about in chapter 1: "I did it on the weekend, when I normally sit around and watch TV," she reported. "Instead, I cleaned my whole apartment"—and lost 3.5 pounds. Of course, fasters should avoid strenuous exercise, but I did recommend a brisk twenty-minute walk or session on a rebounder (a mini trampoline), to help keep their lymph flowing and their blood moving. And I shared with them my own experience during one-day fasts, which always leave me feeling lighter, cleaner, and more energized.

Still, these three clients were a bit skeptical—until the day after the fast. Then they were all smiles. "I wasn't even hungry!" Lucy said triumphantly. "And by the end of the afternoon, I started to feel really good, like I'd somehow gotten free of something."

"I had a little dip in energy around two P.M.," Nila admitted. "But I drank some more juice, and a glass of water, and slowly, I felt my energy flowing back. I ended up feeling calmer, more peaceful, and more focused. It was a very interesting experience."

"Hey, I felt like Superman," Jason remarked. "I don't know what it was, but I felt *strong.*"

I was so pleased that these three Fast Trackers had such a good experience, though I'll admit I wasn't surprised. Healthy fasting—the kind supported by adequate nutritional preparation for the liver and sufficient fiber for the colon—is probably the best-kept secret I know to good health, long-term weight loss, and an overall feeling of well-being. I was thrilled that my three Fast Trackers could share in this wonderful practice, and I'm even more thrilled to be sharing it with you.

So let's get started. Here's the protocol you should follow for your One-Day Detox Diet, followed by an explanation of each element you'll consume and some idea of what you might expect during detox.

THE FAST TRACK ONE-DAY DETOX DIET MIRACLE JUICE PROTOCOL

To conduct your one-day fast, follow this simple, four-step program:

I. PREPARE THE FOLLOWING "MIRACLE JUICE"

2 quarts Cranberry Water (recipe follows)

½ teaspoon ground cinnamon

¼ teaspoon ground ginger

¼ teaspoon ground nutmeg

¾ cup freshly squeezed orange juice

¼ cup freshly squeezed lemon juice

Stevia Plus to taste (2 packets seems ideal)

1. Bring Cranberry Water to a light boil; reduce the heat to low.

2. Place cinnamon, ginger, and nutmeg into a tea ball; add to the Cranberry Water. (For a tangier juice, add the spices directly to the liquid.)

3. Simmer 15 to 20 minutes; cool to room temperature.

4. Stir in the orange and lemon juices. Add Stevia Plus at this time, if desired.

Cranberry Water Recipe

To make 2 quarts (64 ounces), add 8 ounces unsweetened cranberry juice to 56 ounces filtered water OR 3 tablespoons unsweetened cranberry juice concentrate to 60 ounces of filtered water. Recommended brands of unsweetened cranberry juice are Lakewood 100% Organic, Mountain Sun, Trader Joe's, and Knudsen. Recommended brands of unsweetened cranberry juice concentrate are Knudsen and Tree of Life. Be sure to look for juice that has no sugar, corn syrup, or other juices added, including apple or grape.)

II. ALTERNATE DRINKING ONE CUP (8 OUNCES) OF FILTERED WATER AND ONE CUP (8 OUNCES) TO ONE AND A HALF CUPS (12 OUNCES) OF MIRACLE JUICE DURING THE DAY. DRINK AT LEAST 72 OUNCES OF FILTERED WATER THROUGHOUT THE DAY, IN ADDITION TO THE MIRACLE JUICE. MAKE SURE YOU DRINK AT LEAST A CUP OF LIQUID—EITHER THE MIRACLE JUICE OR WATER—EVERY HOUR.

Begin the protocol when you wake up in the morning. A sample day is provided below. You don't have to begin at a specific time, but be sure to have all eight glasses of Miracle Juice in addition to the 72 ounces of water.

6 A.M.	1 cup filtered water
7 A.M.	1 cup Miracle Juice
8 A.M.	1 cup filtered water
9 A.M.	1 cup Miracle Juice
10 A.M.	1 cup filtered water
11 A.M.	1 cup Miracle Juice
12 P.M.	1 cup filtered water
1 P.M.	1 1/2 cups Miracle Juice
2 P.M.	1 cup filtered water
3 P.M.	1 cup Miracle Juice

4 P.M.	1 cup filtered water	
5 P.M.	1 1/2 cups Miracle Juice	
6 P.M.	1 cup filtered water	
7 P.M.	1 cup Miracle Juice	
8 P.M.	1 cup filtered water	
9 P.M.	1 cup Miracle Juice	
10 P.M.	1 cup filtered water	

III. UPON RISING AND AT THE END OF THE DAY TAKE 1 SERVING OF A COLON-CARING SUPPLEMENT, CHOSEN FROM AMONG THE FOLLOWING:

- Powdered Psyllium husks (1 to 2 teaspoons mixed in 8 ounces of water or Miracle Juice)

- Ground or milled flaxseeds (2 to 3 tablespoons mixed in 10 to 12 ounces of water or 8 ounces Miracle Juice)

- Super-GI Cleanse (3 capsules, taken with 10 to 12 ounces of water or 8 ounces Miracle Juice. Available as part of the Fast Detox Diet Kit (see page 83) or individually through Uni-Key at 800-888-4353, or see my Web site, www.fasttrack detox. com.)

IV. ENGAGE ONLY IN LIGHT EXERCISE—EITHER A 20-MINUTE WALK OR 10 MINUTES ON THE REBOUNDER.

(For more on exercise and fitness, see the *Fat Flush Fitness Plan* that I wrote with exercise guru Joanie Greggains.)

A Closer Look at the One-Day Fast

Every ingredient of the One-Day Detox Diet has been specially chosen to stave off hunger; balance your blood sugar; rev up your metabolism; and keep you feeling fit, energized, and trim throughout your fasting day.

The combination of cranberry and citrus juices in the brew is rich in vitamin C, or ascorbic acid. Among its many benefits, ascorbic acid thins and decongests the bile, making it easier for the liver to emulsify (break down) fat at peak efficiency. This combination is also very refreshing and "cleansing" to the palate, offering a satisfying experience that helps mitigate against hunger pangs.

The orange and lemon juices, as we've seen in the Seven-Day Prequel, are key Liver-Loving Foods. Their vitamin C also stimulates the production of glutathione, the major antioxidant on which the liver relies to progress through its two-phase detox process. Vitamin C also helps bind heavy metals and eliminate potentially toxic sulfa drugs.

The cranberry juice helps flush away toxic fluids, which can account for as much as 10 to 15 pounds of water weight trapped in our tissues. This is the water weight that makes us look bloated; it literally weighs us down. Arbutin, a key ingredient in cranberries, is a diuretic that draws both toxins and fluids from our system.

Cranberries are rich in vitamins A, B_1, B_2, B_3, B_5, B_6, C, and E as well as in folic acid, boron, calcium, chromium, copper, iron, magnesium, manganese, molybdenum, phosphorus, potassium, selenium, sodium, and sulfur, all crucial vitamins and minerals for liver activity, as well as for many other bodily functions. These potent red berries are also vital aids to liver detox because they contain exceedingly high levels of lifesaving antioxidants that provide crucial support for both phase 1 and phase 2 detox pathways. Furthermore, their high content of organic acids—such as benzoic, malic, quinic, citric, and ellagic acids—have outstanding therapeutic qualities for many bodily functions. Malic acid, for example, is a potent digestion regulator and helps protect against diarrhea, while ellagic acid has been proven to inhibit the initiation of cancer.

The aromatic spices cinnamon, nutmeg, and ginger all help rev up your metabolism and fight hunger. Several years ago a research team under the guidance of Dr. Richard Anderson discovered that cinnamon contains a flavonoid compound that mimics the body's insulin-regulating activity to control blood sugar metabolism. This is good news, not just for people with type 2 diabetes but also for Fast Trackers. Overproduction of insulin causes your blood sugar to drop quickly, inducing hunger, whereas insulin itself encourages your body to store fat. So cinnamon's natural insulin-like properties will help

THE AMAZING CRANBERRY

Cranberries have so many remarkable benefits, it's hard to know where to start. Since I first began studying this miracle fruit, a host of new cran benefits have come to light. Here's a quick tour:

- Preliminary research suggests that cranberries may be crucial ingredients in cancer prevention. Some researchers believe that cranberries interact positively with two enzymes that either create cancerous cells or help them proliferate. Others have found that cranberries contain elements that may inhibit the growth of colon or prostate cancer cells by protecting our DNA. Still other researchers believe that the quercitin in cranberries may help prevent breast and colon cancer that results from chemicals or toxins or might inhibit the growth of breast-cancer cells.[1]

- New research suggests that elements in cranberries may help prevent atherosclerosis—the buildup of cholesterol, fat, and plaque in the arteries—which is a leading contributor to cardiovascular disease. Scientists have theorized that atherosclerosis begins when low-density lipoprotein (LDL), which you've heard called the "bad" cholesterol, becomes oxidized (affected by oxygen), creating an inflammatory response. This inflammation sets off a chain of events that might lead to arterial lesions and, ultimately, restricted blood flow. Cranberries, however, contain powerful antioxidants that seem to be able to prevent and even reverse this process.[2]

- By the same token, cranberry juice may help raise high-density lipoprotein (HDL), or the "good" cholesterol, according to research presented at the American Chemical Society's annual meeting in April 2004. Dr. Joseph Vinson of the University of Scranton (Pennsylvania) conducted a study suggesting that drinking three glasses of cranberry juice a day might reduce heart disease by 40 percent.[3]

- Although research is still preliminary, some scientists are beginning to explore the possibility that cranberries can help prevent the formation of blood clots and even stroke. Some animal studies also suggest that cranberries can help decrease our body's LDL cholesterol.[4]

- Early research suggests that cranberries might help prevent the formation of ulcers and other gastrointestinal diseases, primarily by inhibiting *Helicobacter pylori*, the bacteria that is implicated in many instances of ulcers and gastrointestinal conditions.[5]

- South African researchers have conducted studies suggesting that cranberry juice may be helpful in preventing kidney stones.[6]

- Cranberries seemed to help experimental subjects resist the effects of *E. coli* bacteria, and so to protect against urinary tract infection. Researchers were especially interested in cranberries' effectiveness against strains of *E. coli* that were resistant to antibiotics.[7]

- Gum disease—the gateway to many other infections—also seems to respond well to the humble cranberry. Dental plaque is a breeding ground for bacteria and other microorganisms that can serve as precursors to a wide range of diseases, including caries (cavities) and periodontal conditions. Cranberry in various forms seems able to help experimental subjects clear the bacteria from their mouths.[8]

- Among the most potent elements in cranberries are *polyphenols*, a kind of plant-based antioxidant that has powerful health-inducing effects. Laboratory studies have shown that eight ounces of cranberry juice contain 567 milligrams of polyphenols—compared to 0.53 milligrams in apple juice and 400 milligrams in red wine. Just two ounces of fresh cranberries contain 373 milligrams of polyphenols, more than much larger servings of oranges, broccoli, blueberries, strawberries, bananas, apples, or white grapes.[9]

keep your blood sugar level throughout the One-Day Detox Diet, which in turn will work to reduce your hunger and cravings.[10] Some researchers even believe that cinnamon is promising as a means of preventing type 2 diabetes.

The warming effects of nutmeg make this spice an aid to digestion, reducing flatulence and helping fight hunger and combat cravings. You may also be interested to know that nutmeg is a powerful aphrodisiac.

Ginger is a peppery and pungent natural vasodilator—a substance that causes the blood vessels to expand. As blood flows more freely through the expanded vessels, your body heat rises and your metabolism revs up along with it. According to an Australian study published in the *International Journal of Obesity*, ginger can cause a metabolic boost of as much as 20 percent, an effect that Anastasia clearly felt when she used her fast day to clean her apartment instead of watching TV as she usually did.[11]

FRESH IS BEST!

Have you ever noticed the way spices tend to pile up in your kitchen for months, sometimes years at a time? It happens to all of us—but the problem is that kept in this way, spices tend to lose their potency. If you've stored them over the stove, the heat sucks away their therapeutic value; if you keep them in the fridge or the freezer, they dry out too quickly. Either way, their health-giving properties evaporate along with their flavor, and much of their benefit is lost.

So for the Miracle Juice, I want you to buy a fresh jar of each spice. Try to find organic and nonirradiated spices. On this detox day, you definitely don't want to add any additional toxins to your body!

Water, of course, helps flush the toxins from our system. It's always important to keep our bodies well hydrated, but it's super-important to do so during a fast. Drinking at least 72 ounces of pure, filtered water along with the juice will keep you feeling refreshed and "full," even as it helps carry the toxins out of your system.

Colon-Caring fiber—whether in the form of psyllium, flaxseed, or Super-GI Cleanse—is the final crucial element of your One-Day Detox Diet. As we've seen, fiber helps scrub your colon clean, breaking down any clogged or impacted fecal matter that might be clinging to your colon walls and ensuring that you won't become constipated or bloated when you resume eating. Fiber also binds with the toxins released during your fast. Think of all the pollutants, additives, and other poisons that might be stored in the 3 to 8 pounds of fat you're going to release on your fasting day, and then make sure you ingest enough fiber to soak them up.

TO WEIGH OR NOT TO WEIGH?

I strongly urge you to weigh yourself only twice during this part of the Fast Track—once on the morning you begin the One-Day Detox Diet, and once at the same time on the following morning. As the day proceeds, you may be tempted to run to the scale and see how it's going—but resist that temptation! Losing weight, particularly as measured in pounds, is not a linear process; it proceeds in an irregular fashion, with sudden drops and occasionally even unexplained increases as your body adjusts to this new regime. Find out your baseline when you begin the one-day fast, and then wait until the next morning to see how you *really* did. Any other numbers that show up along the way will only distort the situation.

Detox Symptoms: Positive and Negative

For most of my Fast Trackers, detox was an extremely positive experience. But for some, particularly those who felt themselves to be dependent on caffeinated drinks, the initial experience of the One-Day

Detox Diet was somewhat uncomfortable. Although many participants reported increased energy, mental clarity, and well-being, some did experience other symptoms, including headaches, fatigue, irritability, foggy thinking, and mild depression.

The explanation is simple: having stored the toxins in our fat, we pay a price for getting rid of them. As we burn up stored body fat for fuel, the oil-soluble toxins we've stored in our fat are also released, sometimes causing distress as they recirculate through the system. If you've been diligent about following the Seven-Day Prequel, and particularly if you've been following the Fat Flush Plan, you may not experience any symptoms at all. But if you do feel tired, grouchy, or headachy, don't lose heart. Realize that these symptoms are an indication that both the fast and the detox process are working and that you'll soon feel even better than you did before.

SKIP THE SUPPLEMENTS

No one is a bigger fan of vitamin, mineral, and nutritional supplements than I am. But one time you should *not* take these otherwise highly recommended products is during a fast. Your body will have a hard time digesting even the finest dietary supplements on an empty stomach, and they might even make you nauseous. You can start taking your supplements again during the Three-Day Sequel, but please skip them during your one-day fast.

Onward and Upward

One of the most powerful aspects of fasting, I've found, is the way it helps you rethink your life and clarify your priorities. I was struck that Lucy, Nila, and Jason all felt re-energized after their One-Day Detox Diet, not only in regard to diet but also as they thought about their lives.

Jason, for example, found himself thinking about how strong the fast had made him feel and when else he had felt that way. He made what I considered a powerful connection, discovering that whenever he was able to extend himself past what he thought were his limits and offer help to family, friends, or colleagues, he experienced that same sense of strength. For him, the One-Day Detox Diet was an opportunity to get in touch with an aspect of his personality that he had often tended to disregard.

Nila spent most of her fast day doing errands and tending to her children, as she had planned. When we first spoke, she described the day as uneventful, though she was relieved that she hadn't experienced either the hunger or the fatigue she had feared. Then she added, "Because I wasn't giving myself food, I started to think about what else I needed during that busy day. Sometimes, I think my needs get lost in all the busy-ness. I don't know what I'll do about that, exactly, but I'm going to think about it."

But it was Lucy who had the most exciting experience. She came bounding into my office, saying triumphantly, "I did it! One whole day without food!" For Lucy, who had always experienced herself as a needy, dependent person, it was liberating to find out that she had more internal resources than she thought. "Besides," she said with a grin, "when I did start eating again, the food tasted *sooooo* good!"

The Miracle Juice was very filling. Only when I had gaps in sipping did I notice a slight want for food. I noticed a slight increase in my energy level, and by the end of the day, the swelling in my ankles had disappeared!
—PATRICIA A. APRE, AGE FIFTY; LOST 5 POUNDS

✳ Warning: Once you have concluded your One-Day Detox Diet, be sure to continue on to chapter 8 and complete the Three-Day Sequel. Fasting without proper follow-up can leave you feeling constipated, bloated, and sluggish, and it can also sabotage your weight loss. Now that you've achieved the hardest part of the program, make sure you seal in your results with the Three-Day Sequel.

YOUR FAST TRACKER LOG:
THE ONE-DAY DETOX DIET

THE MORNING OF THE FAST

MY WEIGHT _____

MY MEASUREMENTS:

WAIST _____

THIGHS _____

THE EVENING OF THE FAST

What strategies worked for me today?

_____

_____

What will I do differently if I ever fast again?

_____

_____

How do I feel about the One-Day Detox Diet?

_____

_____

THE MORNING AFTER THE FAST

MY WEIGHT _____

MY MEASUREMENTS:

WAIST _____

THIGHS _____

Making the Most of Your Day:
Emotional Detox

*Your vision will become clear only when you
look into your heart. Who looks outside, dreams.
Who looks inside, awakens.*
—CARL JUNG

Linda and I had spent several minutes going over the protocol for the Fast Track. An experienced dieter, she wasn't worried about following the Seven-Day Prequel or the Three-Day Sequel. But she was concerned about making it through her One-Day Detox Diet.

"I'm really afraid of how hungry I'll get," she kept saying.

I tried to reassure her, explaining that the Miracle Juice I had created was especially designed to forestall hunger pangs, balance blood sugar, and offer a satisfying, lively taste. I told her about the experiences of other Fast Trackers who had not only avoided feeling hungry but had also enjoyed unexpected surges of energy or benefited from a calm, alert feeling—a steady mental clarity that was the very opposite of the distraction and mental fog that comes from feeling hungry. I even shared my own experiences of one-day fasts. As the day wore on, I told her, I actually felt *less* interested in food, rather than more. I used the day as a kind of sabbath, a day of rest to focus on my feelings, thoughts, and priorities, a time to get clear about what I was really hungry for.

Linda listened politely, but I could see that nothing I said seemed to make much difference. Finally, on impulse, I said, "Linda! What are you really worried about?"

Linda looked at me in distress. "If I'm not eating, what will I *do* with myself all day?" she burst out.

It turned out that Linda, a busy fashion executive, used her weekend mealtimes as a major way to relax and socialize. Although she worked long, grueling hours during the week and spent Saturday on a frantic round of errands (on the rare weekends when she didn't also have to log in some work time), Sunday was a time to power down and hang out with friends. A typical Sunday might start with a leisurely three-hour brunch, followed by drinks with her best friend and then a romantic dinner with her boyfriend. Although Linda didn't necessarily eat very much at any of these meals, she saw them as her only chance to just be. Even when she ate alone, she'd use the time to read, think, and daydream, dawdling for hours in a sidewalk café or at her kitchen table at home.

"Terrific," I said when I heard her explanation. "Then this fast day will have an extra purpose for you. You'll get to find out all the other ways you can 'just be'—ways that have nothing to do with food."

After Linda left, I thought about all the ways the food in our lives is so much more than "just food." I, too, am what my highly respected colleague, counselor, and corporate consultant Linda Spangle calls an "emotional eater," an eloquent phrase that she explains in her breakthrough book *Life Is Hard, Food Is Easy.* I've often used food as comfort, to help me relax, calm me down, or ground me. Some of my warmest memories of family and friends are centered on the holiday meals we've shared or the hours we've spent just hanging out in the kitchen, nurtured by its coziness during those long hard winters when I was living in Bozeman, Montana. And when I want to reach out to a friend in need—someone who's lost a loved one or suffered another tragedy—I turn to the age-old custom of bringing food.

There's nothing wrong with these responses; in fact, I think they're part of what makes us human. But one of the things I love about one-day fasts is the way they help us widen our horizons. Taking a break from eating—while nourishing our bodies with Miracle Juice and drinking lots of pure water—gives us new opportunities to indulge ourselves in other ways. Once we're not using food for comfort, pleasure, and relaxation, we have the chance to find out what other ways we can have fun, pamper ourselves, or enjoy a much-needed break.

Mindful that fasting can be an exciting and perhaps somewhat scary experience for those who have not tried it before, I'm using this chapter to provide you with some emotional and practical support for your fasting day. However you choose to spend it, I know it will be one of your happiest and most satisfying days in a long time. Here are a few suggestions that may make it even better. Browse through them and choose any or all that you think will work for you. Or craft your own special fast day. I wish you luck on your journey!

Conscious Breathing

Conscious breathing is a technique that enables you to become more aware and present with every breath. It's a wonderful way to ground yourself, to relax, to get in touch with your true feelings, or to make a little oasis of calm in the midst of a frantic day. Conscious breathing can be done for as little as two minutes or as much as thirty minutes at a time—while you're stuck in a traffic jam, as part of a lunch hour, or instead of a short nap. On trips to New York, I've even done a bit of conscious breathing in the subway! It's a wonderful way to both calm down and restore your system with energizing oxygen—a nutrient that we are often deprived of in our busy, stressful, shallow-breathing world. If you're concerned about overeating, conscious breathing is a terrific way to begin a meal; take a two- to five-minute "focus time" to connect yourself to your body and release the stress that can interfere with the production of stomach acid, making you more conscious of every bite you take and of how full you are becoming. On today, your fast day, you can indulge in conscious breathing for five minutes at a time to combat hunger pains, or engage in longer sessions as a consciousness-raising experience. Once you master this simple technique, you may start to wonder how you ever got along without it.

COPING WITH HUNGER

The many Fast Trackers who have tried the One-Day Detox Diet reported remarkably few hunger pangs during their time without food. But every so often, you might feel a twinge, whether it's physical hunger or simply the emotional sense that it's time for you to eat. Here are some suggestions to help you make it through those times:

- *Sip some Miracle Juice or water.* The juices and spices in the Miracle Juice will help ease any physical symptoms of hunger you experience, including low blood sugar. Both the juice and the water will help you feel full.

- *Focus on the feeling.* Often, our experience of hunger is an emotional one, linked to powerful feelings of grief, sadness, anger, joy, pleasure, and love. Use one of the conscious breathing exercises, meditations, or suggestions for journal writing given in this chapter to uncover your associations with food and get in touch with your "true" hunger.

- *Give yourself a (nonfood) treat.* Often we become so used to rewarding ourselves, relaxing, or re-energizing with food that we lose track of other means to fill these important needs. Because you're not eating today, you've got lots of time to do other things—so what else might you enjoy? Here are some possibilities—can you think of others?

Conscious Breathing: The Preparation

1. Start by choosing a quiet, peaceful place where you can conduct this exercise. Turn off the radio and the TV and unplug the phone. Just as you are allowing your stomach to be free of food, you will allow your environment to be free of noise—or at least, of noise that makes particular demands on you.

a relaxing walk	only natural oils)
writing in your journal	soaking in the tub, with scented oils and candles
watching a video	
talking to a friend	painting, drawing, molding clay
reading an absorbing book	
getting a manicure, pedicure, or facial	listening to music
	dancing (by yourself is okay)
going for a massage (be sure to ask the masseur to use	doing a crafts project, such as knitting or crocheting[1]

- *Try some conscious breathing.* Deep breathing feeds our bodies with oxygen. If we got more of the "breath of life," I have the feeling none of us would be so hungry. Conscious breathing also expands our awareness of our bodies, and helps us connect to feelings of joy and calm. (I've offered some suggestions for conscious breathing in this chapter.)

- *Meditate.* Similar to conscious breathing, meditation is a way of emptying our minds and allowing our feelings to "flow," rather than getting hung up on what we want and what we'd like to control. Meditation can be a powerful antidote to hunger, because it allows us to experience the sense that we already have everything we need. (You can also find a guide to meditation in this chapter.)

2. Set aside at least five minutes to start. I recommend setting a timer, so that you can focus entirely on your breathing without looking at the clock.

3. Sit in a comfortable position with your feet flat on the floor. Don't lie down—you might fall asleep! Your back should be straight and well supported. The goal is to be alert and present, but relaxed.

Let your hands rest loosely in your lap or on your knees. Don't fold your hands or cross your feet; this exercise works better when each part of your body remains relatively separate.

4. Close your eyes and begin to breathe. Ideally, you should be breathing in on a slow count of eight and breathing out on the same count. If you find it difficult to breathe that slowly, don't worry. Breathe in a slow count of two, and out on two. When you are comfortable with that speed, breathe in on four and out on four. Continue adding time to each inhale and exhale as you feel comfortable, until you've worked your way up to an inhale of eight counts and an exhale of eight counts. If the idea of slowing your breath even further attracts you, go ahead, but eight is slow enough for the exercise to work.

5. Allow your abdomen to expand as your breath fills your diaphragm. Many of us are used to "chest breathing," so that our lungs expand and contract with every breath. That's terrific, but for this exercise you also want to "belly breathe." If you're not sure what this means, place one hand gently on your abdomen. Feel your abdomen expand, like a balloon filling up, as you breathe in. Feel it collapse, like a balloon letting out air, as you breathe out. If you're not used to breathing this way, it may take you a while—even the entire five minutes—to get comfortable with it. Or you may feel comfortable right away. Either way, just take your time and breathe. Don't force your breath. Think of the breath as floating in and floating out. Rather than pushing or pulling, you are simply allowing the breath to enter and leave your body.

Once you're comfortable with the slow, regular belly breathing I've just described, you can begin to allow your consciousness to open as well. You have several choices. You can simply continue to breathe, slowly and calmly, focusing entirely on the process of breathing. Or you can engage in any one of the following journeys. Make a tape of your voice talking you through this process or simply let your own mind guide you.

Conscious Breathing: The Journey

OPTION 1: MY BREATH, MY BODY, MYSELF

I breathe in and feel my breath filling my lungs. I follow my breath as it travels down into my diaphragm. I'm with my breath as it filters into my blood and flows throughout my body. As my breath expands, it fills me all the way up to my skin. When I breathe out, I release everything I do not need. I feel my breath travel inward from my skin, through my blood, back into my diaphragm, up through my lungs. I let it go. Then there is room for a new breath, filling my lungs. I follow my breath as it travels down into my diaphragm . . .

(Continue with this exercise, allowing your awareness of your body to expand with every breath.)

OPTION 2: WHOLE-BODY BREATHING

As I breathe in, I feel the breath begin at the soles of my feet, where they are grounded against the floor. The breath travels up my legs, my thighs, my abdomen, my chest, my shoulders, my throat, my head, and up to the crown of my skull, where I feel it connect to the universe beyond me. Then I release the breath, feeling all tension release with it, down through my face, my neck, my spine, my hips, my thighs, my calves, my ankles, and out through my feet into the ground. When I breathe in again, the breath begins again at the soles of my feet . . .

(Continue with this exercise, allowing your awareness of your body to become more specific with every breath. This is a terrific way to identify and then release tension.)

OPTION 3: BREATHE IN THE GOOD, RELEASE THE BAD

As I breathe in, I draw in [choose an element you would like to connect to; it could be energy, light, love, joy, peace, contentment, or any other positive force or emotion]. I feel [this good thing] moving through my body with the breath. I feel it filling my lungs, my heart, my stomach. I enjoy and savor [this good thing]. As I breathe out, I release [whatever emotion or experience you would like to release, such as fear, worry, anger, confusion, stress, or hunger]. I feel the breath drawing all the [emotion/experience] from my body, from my arms, my legs, my stomach, my head, my chest, my heart. As I breathe out, I release [the emotion/experience] completely. [Continue to repeat this exercise with every breath. This can be an emotional exercise, and I advise you to simply let the emotions flow. If you feel tearful or find yourself beginning to cry, continue to breathe as slowly and evenly as possible, letting the grief flow through you. If you find yourself feeling sudden anger or frustration, experience the feeling while continuing to breathe. I've often noticed that doing this exercise moves me through "negative" emotions to a place of joy and peace, but the key is to allow the emotions to keep flowing. The discipline of a slow, steady breath keeps you safe and grounded while your emotions are released. And if you do find yourself crying, make sure to drink a nice, big glass of water afterward. Nothing is more soothing for your body and spirit.]

Meditation

Meditation is an ancient practice that is part of virtually every religious tradition as well as a technique used by people of no religion. I think meditation is a terrific way to connect to your innermost self, to the thoughts, feelings, and desires that we often bury beneath a mound of busy-ness—or of food! Slowing down long enough to meditate can allow some interesting insights to emerge. It's also a great way to relax and energize yourself at the same time. And I firmly believe that people who meditate regularly have a better chance of making healthy choices about food, since they are more connected to their bodies, feelings, and spirits.

A fast day is a great day to meditate, even for a few minutes. Without the distractions of preparing food, eating it, and then digesting it, you're free to focus on "just being." In fact, many religious traditions combine fasting with meditation, vision quests, and other religious experiences, on the theory that a cleaner, "emptier" body allows more room for spirit. (Many of these religions celebrate eating as well, with feasts and ceremonial foods that follow fasting and prayer.)

Many types of meditation involve "emptying the mind." Other types suggest that you meditate "on" a particular image or topic. If you're interested in learning more about meditation, you might check out your local yoga center, do some research online, or see if you can find a flyer for a class on meditation at your neighborhood health-food store. Here I'll just give you a very preliminary taste of meditation, as one more way to enrich your fasting day.

Meditation: The Preparation

1. Choose a quiet, peaceful place where you won't be interrupted, and unplug the phone. This next portion of time is just for *you*.

2. Set aside at least fifteen minutes to start. Setting a timer will let you focus on your meditation so you don't have to look at the clock.

3. Sit on a chair or sofa, in a comfortable position with your feet flat on the floor. You may have seen meditators sitting cross-legged on the floor, their backs unsupported, and that's terrific; but if this is your first time out, it's more important that you be physically relaxed and comfortable, rather than trying to hold a particular position. Just make sure your back is straight and that your hands and feet are uncrossed.

4. Close your eyes and begin to breathe. It helps to master a bit of conscious breathing as a prequel to meditation, so let me briefly review the principles here. Try breathing in on a slow count of eight and breathing out on the same count. If you can't breathe that slowly right away, start with a count of two, then four, then six, and finally eight.

5. Your goal is to breathe through your belly, allowing your abdomen to expand as your breath fills your diaphragm. If you're

not familiar with this type of breathing, place one hand gently on your abdomen and feel it expand as you breathe in, collapse as you breathe out.

Once you're comfortable with this type of breathing, you can proceed to the meditation itself. I've offered you a few options here, or you can create your own. The goal is to free your mind from its normal round of duties and preoccupations, just as you are freeing your body from its normal focus on eating and digesting.

Meditation: The Journey

OPTION 1: EMPTY YOUR MIND

This is the classic approach to meditation; and although it takes time to master, I think it's well worth it. After all, a technique that wise men and women have been practicing for thousands of years must have something of lasting value to offer!

Basically, your goal is to let your mind empty completely. This can be harder than it sounds, but the process of attempting this practice is worthwhile in itself. Simply continue to breathe in and out, in and out. If a thought or feeling arises, allow it to pass through your mind without holding onto it. Think of yourself as watching the thought as it passes through your mind. You might say to yourself, "I am thinking about my job," or "I am feeling anxious." If you choose this approach, let your descriptions of your thoughts be as specific as possible, "I am thinking about Melanie and the way she ignored me at the office on Thursday. I am feeling anxious about Melanie. I am wondering if she doesn't like me anymore." Becoming conscious of each thought or feeling in this way can be very helpful in letting them pass.

I believe that if we learn to let our thoughts and feelings pass through us, easily and lightly, we'll also have an easier time digesting our food, absorbing what's good and nutritious and releasing what's toxic and unnecessary. So let this time of meditation be a time of "eating," "digesting," and then "releasing" thoughts.

Option 2: Meditate on Hunger

As you breathe, direct your thoughts, emotions, and physical sensations to focus on hunger. Again, don't push your thoughts in any particular direction or try to control your feelings or sensations. Just hold the word *hunger* in your mind and see what springs up around it.

When I did this exercise recently, I was surprised at the flow of apparently unconnected thoughts and feelings that passed through my mind. I found myself thinking of childhood memories, recent experiences, and some events that happened quite early in my career as a nutritionist. I also felt many emotions glide through me: fear, anger, grief, intense physical hunger, and then a sense of peace and calm. I ended the exercise with a remarkable feeling of fullness, as though I had just eaten the most delicious and satisfying meal.

Each of us is different, of course, and your journey on this meditation will likely be quite different from mine. But if hunger is an issue in your life, this may be a useful way to explore your relationship to it in a new and exciting way.

Option 3: Meditate on Satisfaction

This exercise allows you to explore the other side of the coin—the experience of feeling satisfied and "full." I've noticed in my practice that while it's often easy for us to talk about hunger, we frequently shy away from talking about what satisfies us. Could it be that feeling "full" is sometimes scarier or more disturbing than feeling hungry? Might it be hard to let ourselves feel truly satisfied if someone we love is going hungry, spiritually or emotionally or in some other way? Or maybe we're so preoccupied with what we have to accomplish next that we've simply lost the habit of slowing down and feeling "finished," satisfied, happy with our day's work.

As you can see, satisfaction offers a rich field of exploration for your meditation—and a particularly interesting one for a fasting day. I invite you to explore this issue and see what comes up for you. You may be in for a surprise!

VISUALIZATION

Visualizing yourself in a given situation and then watching yourself move through the experience can be a powerful way to learn more about who you are, how you feel, and what you want. A fast day can be a particularly useful day for visualizing. Because you are already trying something new, why not put yourself mentally into another new or unusual situation and see what happens?

If you're interested in exploring this technique, I've included some suggestions and some visualizations that you might use in Appendix B.

Keeping a Journal

I love writing in my journal! It's a time to unwind, to get in touch with myself, to learn things about myself that I didn't even know I knew. I've always advocated journal writing as an integral part of my weight-loss plans, because I believe that only when we're really aware of who we are and what we want can we make the healthy food choices that our bodies and spirits need.

If you simply want to grab your journal and write for a few minutes, more power to you! If you'd like a bit of guidance, see page 124 for a sample journal page to get you started.

FLOWER REMEDIES

I couldn't let this chapter end without sharing with you one other invaluable support. The Bach Flower Remedies are an extraordinary noninvasive set of thirty-eight natural flower essences that help you cope with a wide range of challenging and sometimes difficult emotions, such as might arise during a fast day, or at any other stressful time of your life. If you'd like to use any of these marvelous harmonizers, what I have come to call "psychotherapy in a bottle," check out Appendix C.

The End . . . and the Beginning

When I next saw Linda, she was almost glowing with excitement. Her fast day, she told me, had been a revelation. Although at first she felt anxious and frustrated at the prospect of going without her daily meals, she was determined to stick it out. She had even planned a day of being entirely alone, so she could "fully experience the fast."

"I thought I would be so bored," she said in amazement. "And I'll admit it—for the first couple of hours, I was. I was kind of pacing my apartment, wishing I'd made other plans. But then I thought, 'Well, just because I'm fasting doesn't mean I have to stay home.' I ended up going for a walk, browsing in my neighborhood bookstore, and dropping by the local crafts store. On impulse, I actually picked up a set of watercolors. I went home, set up a big bowl of fruit—and started to paint it!" She laughed. "If I couldn't *eat* food, I guess I had to do something *else* with it."

Although Linda didn't expect ever to take painting seriously, she was happy just to recall that she had once enjoyed this pastime in college and that she had lots of talents and interests that weren't encompassed by her current job or her current friends. "I love my job, I love my boyfriend, and my friends are the best," she told me. "But I think I'd gotten just a little too stuck in a rut. This fast day was a real wake-up call that there were things I might be hungry for that I was ignoring." When she left my office, I knew that Linda's journey of exploration was just beginning.

> *My complexion is better, and I had a wonderful sleep last night. I learned more about myself, and how I can eat to feel better about myself. I would definitely do this again because it's a terrific detox and my body feels so good today. And this is just the first day!*
>
> —CRYSTAL FRASER, TWENTY-SIX; LOST 5.5 POUNDS

YOUR FAST TRACKER JOURNAL:
YOUR FASTING DAY

Now that I've begun my fast, I realize that

_____

_____

_____

_____

Right now, I'm feeling

_____

_____

_____

_____

Something I didn't expect to learn from fasting was

_____

_____

_____

I will make use of what I learned today by

_____

_____

_____

Sealing in the Results:
The Three-Day Sequel

*The reward for work well done is
the opportunity to do more.*
—Jonas Salk

✳ Warning: You *must* follow the One-Day Detox Diet with this
Three-Day Sequel, or your re-entry into normal eating might
leave you more bloated, constipated, and "toxic" than you were
before. Fasting without follow-up support means that the toxins
released into your bloodstream during the fast may remain in
your system, making you feel tired, anxious, headachy and more
fatigued than when you started. You'll also be likely to gain more
weight.

THE FAST TRACK SEQUEL—THREE DAYS

Seal in the results of your one-day fast with the eight simple steps that are described here.

I. EACH DAY, CHOOSE AT LEAST ONE OF THE FOLLOWING PROBIOTIC FOOD SOURCES TO RESTORE "FRIENDLY BACTERIA":

- sauerkraut (½ cup): You can either make your own sauerkraut or buy an organic, raw variety. Most store-bought sauerkraut is processed with heat, which kills the naturally occurring enzymes and microflora; so check the label very carefully.

- yogurt (1 cup): Nonfat, low-fat, and whole-milk yogurt are all fine, but look for plain yogurt whose label reads "active and live active cultures."

II. BEGINNING ON DAY TWO, TAKE 1 OR MORE TABLETS OF HYDROCHLORIC ACID IN A FORMULA THAT CONTAINS AT LEAST 500 TO 550 MILLIGRAMS OF BETAINE HYDROCHLORIDE WITH AT LEAST 130 MILLIGRAMS OF PEPSIN, AND 50 MILLIGRAMS OF OX BILE EXTRACT, BEFORE EACH MEAL. (SEE "RESOURCES.")

III. EACH DAY, CHOOSE AT LEAST ONE LIVER-LOVING FOOD FROM EACH GROUP:

1. **The Crucifers (½ cup cooked or 1 cup raw, about the size of a small fist)**
   cabbage, cauliflower, Brussels sprouts, broccoli, broccoli sprouts

2. **Green Leafy Vegetables and Herbs (½ cup cooked or 1 cup raw)**
   parsley, kale, watercress, chard, cilantro, beet greens, collards, escarole, dandelion greens, mustard greens

3. Citrus (1 orange or juice of 1/2 a lemon or lime)

   orange, lemon, lime

4. Sulfur-Rich Foods

   garlic (at least one clove, minced), onions (1/2 cup cooked), eggs (2), daikon radish (1/4 cup sliced, either raw or cooked)

5. Liver Healers

   artichoke (1 small artichoke or 4 cooked artichoke hearts), asparagus (1/2 cup cooked), beets (1/2 cup cooked or 1 cup raw), celery (2 medium stalks), dandelion root tea (1 to 2 cups), whey (1 to 2 scoops), nutritional yeast flakes (1 to 2 teaspoons)

IV. EACH DAY, CHOOSE AT LEAST TWO OF THE FOLLOWING COLON-CARING FOODS

powdered psyllium husks (1 to 2 teaspoons in 8 ounces of water), milled or ground flaxseeds (2 to 3 tablespoons), The Super-GI Cleanse (3 capsules, taken with 10 to 12 ounces of water) (see p. 215), carrot (1 small raw), apple (1 small raw with skin), pear (1 small raw with skin), berries (1 cup)

V. EACH DAY, DRINK HALF YOUR BODY WEIGHT IN OUNCES OF FILTERED OR PURIFIED WATER.

VI. EACH DAY, MAKE SURE YOU HAVE AT LEAST TWO SERVINGS (THE SIZE OF THE PALM OF YOUR HAND) OF PROTEIN IN THE FORM OF LEAN BEEF, VEAL, LAMB, SKINLESS CHICKEN, TURKEY, OR FISH, OR, IF YOU'RE A VEGAN OR VEGETARIAN, AT LEAST 2 TABLESPOONS A DAY OF A HIGH-QUALITY BLUE-GREEN ALGAE OR SPIRULINA SOURCE.

VII. EACH DAY, MAKE SURE YOU HAVE 1 TO 2 TABLESPOONS OF OIL IN THE FORM OF OLIVE OIL, FLAXSEED OIL, OR THE WOMAN'S OIL (A FLAXSEED OIL–BLACK CURRANT SEED OIL BLEND).

VIII. Avoid the following Detox Detractors:

- *Excess fat,* especially trans fats from margarine and processed and fried foods

- *Sugar and all its relatives,* including high-fructose corn syrup, honey, molasses, maple syrup, sugar cane crystals, pure sugar cane juice, evaporated cane juice, dried cane juice, maltodextrin, and all products ending in "-ose" (such as sucrose, dextrose, fructose, and levulose)

- *Artificial sweeteners,* including aspartame, sucralose or Splenda, and sugar alcohols (such as maltitol, mannitol, sorbitol, and xylitol)

- *Refined carbohydrates,* including white rice and products made from white flour

- *Gluten,* found in wheat, rye, barley, and all their products (including breads, pastas, crackers, and crusts); also found in many "low-carb" products (such as packaged cereals, macaroni and cheese, pizza dough mix, spaghetti, shells, tortillas, pancake/waffle mixes, and cookies) and in vegetable proteins, modified food starch, some soy sauces, and distilled vinegars

- *Soy protein isolates,* found in low-carb "energy" bars and soy protein powders; and processed soy foods (such as soy milk, soy cheese, soy ice cream, soy hot dogs, and soy burgers)

- *Alcohol; over-the-counter drugs; and caffeine,* including coffee, tea, sodas, and chocolate

- *Mold,* found on overly ripe fruits, especially melons, bananas, and tropical fruits

Sealing in the Results of Your Fast

Miriam was a short, intense woman in her early fifties who had struggled with weight loss since she'd gone into early menopause in her mid-forties. When she heard about the Fast Track, she was thrilled, particularly after I suggested that its special Seven-Day Prequel, Miracle Juice, and Three-Day Sequel might actually rev up her metabolism and make it easier for her to keep the weight off.

Miriam had no problem following the Seven-Day Prequel—an intelligent and well-read person, she well understood the need for supporting the liver and colon before beginning a fast. And when she lost 5 pounds on her One-Day Detox Diet, she was delighted.

Then came the Three-Day Sequel. Happy with the results she'd already enjoyed, Miriam decided to skip the follow-up to the fast. When I saw her a week later, she had gained back half the weight she'd lost, and she was suffering from constipation and bloating. I asked her about how closely she'd followed the Fast Track protocol. Blushing, she admitted that she'd failed to complete the Three-Day Sequel.

"I felt like I was done," she told me. "I didn't really see the need to keep going."

Because she was already so frustrated and uncomfortable, I didn't have the heart to scold her. I gave her some suggestions for adding fiber to her diet, and sent her on her way. But her experience reminded me just how important it is to give yourself the proper nutritional support *after* your fast as well as before. Undergoing the Fast Track is a wonderful opportunity to unclog your colon and begin detoxing your system. But if you don't follow up with extra colon and liver support—and particularly with extra fiber to bind the toxins you have released through your weight loss—you could end up in worse shape than before you began.

So let's take a closer look at the Three-Day Sequel. As I hope you've realized by now, every single step of this program is there for a reason—to support your weight loss and your health. If you skip any aspect of the program, you'll only be cheating yourself.

Ease Back into Eating

My first suggestion is that you ease back into eating by choosing cooked, low-fat foods that are easy to digest. For breakfast, for example, try the Morning-After Puffy Apple Flaxcake (page 203). This

TAKE IT SLOW AND EASY

Keep in mind that how you break the fast is just as important as the fast itself. And the way you eat is just as important as what you eat. So, first and foremost, because digestion begins in the mouth, you must eat slowly and chew your food very well. Try to chew about thirty times per bite.

Of course, you shouldn't overeat—less is more when you're breaking a fast. And make your transition into your postfast eating by sticking with light and easy-to-digest foods as well as focusing on cooked foods rather than raw (it's easier on the digestion).

Finally, keep the food combinations simple. Use this time as an opportunity to appreciate how good food tastes when you haven't eaten for an entire day and how nourishing your new food choices will be for your 3 trillion cells.

recipe contains high-fiber flaxseed and pectin-rich apple, which both bind up toxic wastes and help elimination. If possible, have this pancake for breakfast your first day—or even all three days of the Sequel to get things moving. (You will note that the Morning-After Puffy Apple Flaxcake already contains two sources of fiber, so you may not need to choose an additional fiber source that day. Or you might—you will know by how you feel.)

You might also break the fast with easy-to-digest soups like A Cabbage Soup for All Seasons (page 185), steamed veggies like Brussels Sprouts à l'Orange (page 187), or lightly sautéed greens like Garlicky Greens with Ginger and Lemon (page 188). To keep it even simpler, try plain old scrambled eggs with some cilantro for one of your meals. Or make a meal of baked chicken brushed with lemon juice and garlic or grilled fish with any one of my special salads, such as Firecracker Slaw (page 184).

In any case, keep your choices very basic, especially for the first day. Go for foods in simple combinations. Don't eat fruits and vegetables in the same meal because these foods require different sets of enzymes to digest, and after a fast, that can cause *in*digestion in sensitive systems. You should also choose just one protein per meal. This could be accompanied by a soup or some steamed or pureed veggies. Save your fruit to eat by itself, as a snack.

I've suggested this transition period as a safeguard to your health. But you might also want to use this time to savor the smells, tastes, and textures of the food you eat. Choose foods with bright, rich colors, such as steamed red peppers, yellow squash, and purple cabbage. Besides being pleasing to the eye, the intense color also indicates the presence of *flavonoids*, powerful antioxidants that will both nourish your liver and fight the aging process. Keep your portions small, especially for the first day. This is an opportunity to discover how much—or how little—you need to feel full, particularly when you are savoring every bite.

Making Friends with Bacteria

You've already noticed that I started this Three-Day Sequel by instructing you to consume probiotics in the form of sauerkraut or yogurt, fermented foods that will help restore friendly bacteria to your system. The use of these probiotic fermented foods is perhaps one of the most important, and most overlooked, aspects of nutrition, and one that will be a particular problem for any of you who've been on a low-carb, high-protein diet. Whenever you eat heavy-duty amounts of protein and cheese from nonorganically raised animals, you are unknowingly ingesting secondhand antibiotics that are contained in all conventionally farmed beef, chicken, or pork—antiobiotics that are equal-opportunity drugs and kill off all of your bacteria, too, even the friendly ones on which your body depends.

As we saw in chapter 3, our intestinal tracts are full of "friendly bacteria" whose job is to help us digest our food and to combat the unfriendly bacteria that cause disease. In our large bowel alone, some 100 trillion bacteria make their home, including more than 400 different species. They actually weigh about 3 pounds, but that's one type of weight you don't want to lose. Without these friendly flora, you couldn't synthesize vitamins, break down toxins, or digest fiber—they're the ones that break down indigestible plant materials into the short-chain fatty acids on which your colon cells desperately rely. They also help transport nutrients, produce lactase and other enzymes to help you digest milk sugars, and help in the synthesis of vitamin K and all the B vitamins.

Your liver is also happy when friendly bacteria are flourishing, because some research indicates that a shortage of beneficial bacteria is correlated with cirrhosis and diabetes. And new studies suggest that friendly bacteria may offer a host of other benefits, including helping you digest fats, proteins, and carbohydrates, and controlling excess LDL or "bad" cholesterol levels.

The weight-loss advantage of such elements is clear. But perhaps most useful of all for your weight loss is understanding that when your body is finally digesting and absorbing nutrients at peak efficiency, you won't be nearly so hungry. You'll be able to eat far less food, with far greater satisfaction.

WHICH ARE THE GOOD BACTERIA?

If you're welcoming the friendly bacteria into your system, you should probably know them by name! The two main categories are called *lactobacillus* and *bifido* bacterium. The lactobacilli hang out in your small intestines, while the bifido bacteria live in the large intestines. These tiny organisms prevent damage to the lining of your gastrointestinal tract and help crowd out the really bad or pathogenic bacteria (like the infamous *Escherichia coli*) by creating a "barrier wall" in your intestines. By keeping in check disease-causing microbes, probiotics are your immune system's best friends. These good bacteria may also be the newest weapon in the fight against cancer, balancing glucose and lipid levels and helping ward off osteoporosis.

Good vs. Bad Bacteria:
A Balance of Power

Your small intestine is the home of 60 percent of your immune system, which literally resides in the lining of this key organ. When you consider that for most of human history, the biggest dangers to our health would have come from eating poisonous food, it makes sense that our bodies are designed for a quick first-line response whenever something unhealthy enters our intestinal tract. This immune response largely depends on good bacteria—another reason why it's so important to promote their growth.

The problem, of course, comes from the fact that many of the same conditions friendly to good bacteria also provide a breeding ground for bad bacteria and other life forms, including parasites and yeast. And, by the same token, the antibiotics (literally, "anti-life" medications) that destroy bad bacteria and the treatments that rid you of yeast infections are also likely to kill off good bacteria.

In the healthy intestinal system, good bacteria, bad bacteria, and yeast create a kind of balance of power, in which all three life forms live within you, with the good bacteria free to do its healthy work. Ideally, you want a ratio of 85 percent friendly bacteria to 15 percent unfriendly bacteria. Killing off the good bacteria upsets the balance of power in your internal ecology, however, leaving room for the yeast to get out of control, with such symptoms as bloating, gas, diarrhea, eczema, hives, and even psoriasis.[1]

If you've been taking antibiotics, you need to make extra sure that you're also taking *probiotics* at the same time and for at least two months thereafter to restore the balance of bacterial power. By the same token, now that you've completed two thirds of the Fast Track, you need to replenish your friendly bacteria. By detoxifying your system—particularly if you were successful at freeing your colon from any fecal encrustation that built up along its walls—you've also made life far more difficult for the friendly bacteria within your gut. So in this Three-Day Sequel, we're going to start building up those helpful bacteria. This is where both sauerkraut (fermented cabbage) and yogurt (fermented milk) come into the health picture.

Sauerkraut is a natural source of lactic acid, a highly beneficial organic acid that results from the fermentation or culturing of foods. Of all the organic acids formed during the fermentation process, lactic acid is the most powerful inhibitor of the type of bacteria that causes putrefaction in the gut; yet it never makes your system overly acid.

Sauerkraut is such a healing food that during the Civil War, when the "soured cabbage" was added to prisoners' diets, smallpox death rates plummeted from 90 percent to only 5 percent. Although you probably don't have to worry about smallpox today, you can imagine the beneficial effect of this common food on the nasty bacteria in your own system. Sauerkraut is a rich source of *Lactobacillus plantarum*, a potent strain of friendly bacteria that gives *Candida, Salmonella, E. coli*, and parasites the heave-ho.

You can make your own vitamin-, fiber-, and enzyme-rich sauerkraut (see Ann Louise's Homemade Sauerkraut on page 204), or buy

THE FAST TRACK PROBIOTIC WAY

If you are still not a sauerkraut fan, even after you've tried the fabulous Sauerkraut Stuffed Tomatoes (page 205), and if yogurt isn't your idea of high-culture cuisine—not even a Fruity Yogurt snack (page 206)—you do have two supplement options for your probiotics:

- Flora-Key (1 teaspoon once daily in liquid)

  This powdered probiotic contains a basic combination of lactobacillus, bifidobacterium, and fructooligosaccharides (FOS), from complex sugars that function as a "prebiotic," a food that feeds the beneficial bacteria while discouraging harmful bacteria. Both the lactobacillus (which mainly resides in the small intestines) and the bifidobacterium (which is most predominant in the large intestines) help normalize overall bowel function and ferment fiber, which creates short-chain fatty acids that feed the colon. (Note: This supplement is contained in the Fast Detox Diet Kit. See page 83.)

it ready-made in your local health-food store. But again, make sure that the sauerkraut you buy is raw because cooking sauerkraut kills the enzymes and microflora that you need to restore the friendly bacteria. The Rejuvenative Foods brand is one to buy.

Yogurt is also a tried and true food source of probiotics, chock full of lactobacilli, but only if it's made with live active cultures. It's been used for centuries to help digestive problems, stop diarrhea, enhance immunity, and fight off infection because of its high content of the lactobacilli and *L. thermophilus* strain of friendly bacteria. Cow, goat, and sheep yogurt are all available and each is a healthy choice, but steer clear of frozen yogurt—freezing kills the live cultures. Make sure whatever yogurt you buy says "made with active and live cultures" on the label. My favorite brands include Nancy's and Horizon, both of which you can count on for multifaceted probiotic action.

- Dr. Ohhira's Probiotics 12 Plus (5 capsules in the morning on an empty stomach and 5 capsules before bedtime).

  This is the world's best-selling probiotic supplement—and for good reason. It contains twelve strains of viable lactic acid bacteria, four organic acids, twelve amino acids, eight minerals, ten vitamins, naturally developed FOS, hydrogen peroxide, and bacteriocins. It also contains the only known strain of lactic acid bacteria (the TH10 strain from tempeh) that has clinically been shown to neutralize antibiotic-resistant superbugs *E. coli* and *H. pylori*—the bacteria responsible for most ulcers, migraine headaches, glaucoma, acid reflux, and even rosacea. Scientists have established that the lactic acid bacteria contained in Dr. Ohhira's probiotic product are 6.25 times stronger than any naturally occurring lactic acid bacteria.

  If you wish to continue taking this formula past the Three-Day Sequel, use this "5 and 5" protocol for the first week and then switch to a "2 and 2" regime.

Tip: Apple cider vinegar contains acids that support friendly bacteria in their fight against yeast, even as it cleanses your digestive system. Apple cider vinegar also has a long history as a folk remedy. You could actually make your own—it's nothing but fresh-pressed apple juice allowed to ferment over four to six weeks at room temperature—but it's easier to buy raw, unfiltered vinegar and add it to salad dressings or to give your veggies a little zing. Some research suggests that it helps remove calcium deposits from joints and blood vessels without affecting the calcium levels in your bones and teeth. It's also rich in potassium. You can even use it to disinfect wounds or abrasions. Look for certified organic apple cider vinegar. Commercial or "natural" ciders may be diluted with meta-bisulfite. A brand I like is Bragg's (available in most health-food stores throughout the country), because I know they don't use anything but apples.

Helpful Hydrochloride

Now that you've cleansed so many toxic wastes from your system, you need to make sure that no more toxins accumulate from putrefying proteins or undigested food. A little HCl taken before meals will help your stomach acids do their job—a particularly necessary supplement if you've been on a low-carb diet, which, as we saw in chapter 3, tends to overload your system with proteins that deplete your stomach acids. One of the nice things about adding HCl is that it's one of the very few inorganic acids that is a normal constituent of the body anyway, so you can't lose by adding a bit more. And if there's extra ox bile in your HCl supplement, as I recommend, you'll get a boost in digesting fat and promoting peristalsis, that undulating motion in the small intestine that leads to proper elimination. To find out whether you need to add this vital supplement to your daily diet, take the Hydrochloric Challenge (page 50) and follow the recommendations accordingly. Wait until the second day of the Sequel to begin taking your HCl supplement. Starting too soon after fasting could cause nausea or discomfort. Remember, I recommend a supplement that includes 500 to 550 milligrams of betaine hydrochloride, 150 milligrams of pepsin, and 65 milligrams of ox bile.

Fun with Fiber

As we've seen, keeping your fiber content high is super-important in this Three-Day Sequel. You need fiber to bind up the toxins you've released and to keep food moving through your system. I strongly recommend the Morning-After Apple Flaxcake (page 203) for your first breakfast as a food source that includes both soluble and insoluble fiber—and is light and filling, to boot. You may enjoy it so much that you have it all three days! And because this breakfast dish is so fiber rich, you don't need to choose any other fiber source for that day.

It's especially important to chew fibrous foods slowly and carefully. If you're getting your fiber in the form of apples, carrots, celery, or berries, make sure you chew each bite thoroughly. You can try counting to twenty-five on every chew before you swallow. Or simply focus on the amazing tastes that are released into your mouth with every bite. For these post-fast meals, try not to do anything while you eat except focus on the food—no reading, watching TV, or even talking. Concentrate on the delicious sensations that even the humblest meal can offer you, and marvel at Nature's bounty of fruits, vegetables, herbs, and spices.

Don't Forget the Water!

By now you've been drinking so much water, you may feel as though you're ready to float away! But don't stop drinking. You really need the excess fluids to keep the toxins flowing *out* of your body, as well as to keep food moving through your bowels. The worst possible time to cut back on water is in the three days after a fast—that's when your system needs more lubrication than ever, particularly because you are also keeping up your fiber intake, which can have a dehydrating effect.

Looking toward the Next Level

Now that you've completed your time on the Fast Track, I hope you've both lost some weight and gained a new attitude. I'll make a small confession here: I didn't want you to try detox just for the eleven days it took to complete the Fast Track. My real agenda was for you to become so hooked on detox that you'd start to eat healthy, clean, organic foods; cleanse your system regularly; and discover that the best way to lose weight and to keep it off is to protect your health, your body, and our planet.

What you'll do from here is up to you. But if you'd like some guidance on how to take the Fast Track to the next level, read on. Chapter 9 will offer you everything you need to know—whether you're looking for another quick fix after your next holiday splurge, or a lifelong devotion to clean, healthy, and delicious food.

> *Usually I'm tired and don't get much done at home. But on my fast day, I took a long, slow walk, then cleaned house and did five loads of wash. "Wow," I said to myself. "It's 11:45 at night and I'm not tired yet." At lunch, I wasn't hungry even after my daughter ate a double cheeseburger and fries right in front of me. Wow!!! I plan on using your One-Day Detox Diet again— because it works! I love not feeling tired all day. I feel rejuvenated and more focused. I love the abundance of energy—and I love seeing my chin back.*
>
> —BEVERLY GRZEJKA, FIFTY-SEVEN; LOST 4.25 POUNDS

YOUR FAST TRACKER LOG: THE SEQUEL

DAY ONE

I. The probiotics I ate today

1. _____

Others: _____

II. The Liver-Loving Foods I ate today

1. _____

2. _____

3. _____

4. _____

5. _____

Others: _____

III. The Colon-Caring Foods I ate today

1. _____

2. _____

Others: _____

IV. The water I drank today

I need to drink _____ ounces.

Today I drank _____ ounces of water.

V. Today I did/did not avoid all Detox Detractors.

My evaluation

How do I feel about how I stuck to the Fast Track today?

_____

_____

_____

What strategies worked for me?

_____

_____

_____

What will I do differently tomorrow?

_____

_____

_____

DAY TWO

I. The probiotics I ate today

1. _____

Others: _____

II. The Liver-Loving Foods I ate today

1. _____

2. _____

3. _____

4. _____

5. _____

Others: _____

III. The Colon-Caring Foods I ate today

1. _____

2. _____

Others: _____

IV. The water I drank today

I need to drink _____ ounces.

Today I drank _____ ounces of water.

V. Today I did/did not avoid all Detox Detractors.

My evaluation

How do I feel about how I stuck to the Fast Track today?

_____

_____

_____

What strategies worked for me?

_____

_____

_____

_____

What will I do differently tomorrow?

_____

_____

_____

DAY THREE

I. The probiotics I ate today:

1. _____

Others:: _____

II. The Liver-Loving Foods I ate today:

1. _____

2. _____

3. _____

4. _____

5. _____

Others: _____

III. The Colon-Caring Foods I ate today:

1. _____

2. _____

Others: _____

IV. The water I drank today

I need to drink _____ ounces.

Today I drank _____ ounces of water.

V. Today I did/did not avoid all Detox Detractors.

My evaluation

How do I feel about how I stuck to the Fast Track today?

_____

_____

_____

What strategies worked for me?

_____

_____

_____

_____

What will I do differently tomorrow?

_____

_____

_____

Taking It to the Next Level:

Enzymes, Nucleotides, and Your Detox Diet for Life

If you can find a path with no obstacles,
it probably doesn't lead anywhere.
—FRANK A. CLARK

As I think about the dieters who've tried the Fast Track so far, three people in particular keep coming to mind.

Jewelle ended her Fast Track experience totally jazzed about organic food, regular detox, and healthy eating. "I always knew that the environment was important," she told me with characteristic enthusiasm. "But I never really got how much it was affecting me. I can see already how detox and organic food is going to keep the weight off—and that's terrific. But I can also see how much better I feel when I'm eating better. I have more energy, my mind is clear, and I feel ready to take on the world. Now that I feel so terrific, I can't imagine going back to the way I was before."

Mercedes had a completely different perspective. "Look, I'm glad I lost a few pounds," she said bluntly. "And frankly, I do feel better.

But I'll tell you right now, if I can't have dessert a few times a month, and if I have to watch every bite that goes into my mouth to make sure it's organic, I'll go nuts. Life isn't worth living when you're that careful. I'd love to do another detox sometime. But I don't want to go crazy."

Jason had yet another way of looking at his Fast Track experience. "Doing the detox was really wild," he told me. "I didn't know I'd feel so much better, just from that one day without food. I was already doing Fat Flush, though, and I really like Fat Flush. So what I want to know is, how does Fast Track fit with Fat Flush?"

Become Your Own Nutritionist

As I thought about these dieters, I realized that I needed to provide three more pieces of the puzzle to help them—and you—stay on the Fast Track:

1. First, I have to tell you about some breakthrough dietary elements whose importance I've recognized for quite some time: *enzymes* and *nucleotides*. No matter what you decide to eat or how you organize your diet, you must include foods that contain these vital substances that maximize your energy, slow down the aging process, and promote longevity. You'll be amazed at the dramatic difference they can make in both your weight loss and your health.

2. Next, I'll share with you what I know about how to make your diet as clean as possible. Here's my philosophy in a nutshell: *When you can, buy organic. When you can't, make the healthiest choices you can.* Did you realize that the most popular fruits in America are also the most toxic? Apples, peaches, pears, strawberries, and raspberries are sprayed with more pesticides than any other fruits. So if you can't afford organic apples, or if organic strawberries (fresh or frozen) aren't available in your local supermarket, have a plum instead of an apple, and choose blueberries instead of strawberries. I'll talk you through simi-

lar choices for red meat, poultry, fish, dairy products, and vegetables, helping you choose the cleanest, healthiest foods to support your new commitment to detox.

3. Finally, I'll give you three different approaches to a Fast Track Detox Diet for Life, so you can choose the one that works best for your temperament and lifestyle. For people like Jewelle, who want to kick things up a notch and pursue the purest possible diet and lifestyle, I've developed Path A, "the Fastest Track." For folks like Mercedes, who want to indulge every now and then, I've come up with Path B, "the Cheater's Diet." And for dieters like Jason, who want to rely on Fast Flush but to also benefit from one-day fasts, I've developed Path C, "the Fast Track Mix and Match."

As you can see, this is a somewhat different approach from what you'll find in most other diet books, which tend to insist you follow only a single path. I don't think that any one approach meets the needs of everybody. But I do think that everyone needs to know how to make the healthiest possible choices. So in this chapter, I give you the tools to become your own nutritionist. My guidance, advice, and twenty-five years of experience as nutritionist and researcher are at your disposal!

So let's get started. I can't wait to tell you about enzymes and nucleotides, which I consider among the major nutritional building blocks for the twenty-first-century diet.

Beyond Vitamins and Minerals— The Enzyme Connection

FAST TRACK MAINSTAY: I CUP OF SPROUTS OR ONE BLENDED SALAD PER DAY FOR LIVING ENZYMES

Enzyme nutrition represents a whole new arena in the world of health and healing. It was first popularized by Dr. Edward Howell in his groundbreaking 1986 work, *Enzyme Nutrition*. I'm delighted to share with you here a way of incorporating this nutritional element into your daily diet.

Enzyme is the scientific term for a living catalyst—an element that acts within our bodies to enable a chemical reaction. I like to think of enzymes as living sparkplugs, vital catalysts that fire up our life force, because without the thousands of enzymes working within our system, none of the biochemical processes on which our lives depend could occur. Found in every one of our cells, enzymes are what make it possible for vitamins, minerals, and hormones to affect our bodies. And they play a key role in our digestion.

Because of their therapeutic value, enzymes have been used to treat a whole host of diseases, from arthritis and autoimmune disorders to sports injuries and viral infections. Enzymes also combat cancer in a variety of ways while helping reduce the inflammatory response that many cutting-edge researchers now see as a major factor in cancer, cardiovascular problems, and autoimmune conditions.[1]

Decreased enzyme activity has been correlated with digestive difficulties, lethargy—and weight gain. Besides keeping us slim and trim, enzymes also help keep us young. In fact, Nobel Prize–winning chemist James Sumner, M.D., claimed way back in 1946 that the "middle-aged feeling" of sluggishness and creeping age was the result of our bodies' reduced enzyme levels. His insight is supported by research associating decreased enzyme activity with such chronic conditions as skin disease, allergies, diabetes, and cancer.[2]

If lower enzyme levels are associated with aging, adding enzymes to your diet will put a sparkle in your eye and add a glow to your skin. You'll feel younger and more energetic as you increase your enzyme intake, and you may even notice fewer wrinkles, not to mention better digestion. Because enzymes rev up your system to work so efficiently, they support detox—particularly liver detox—and they contribute to weight loss.

Enzymes have their foes, however, many of them the same Detox Detractors we've come to know so well. Enzyme Enemies include first and foremost the cooking process itself. Joining the ranks are carcinogens, fluoride (found in our water supply), exposure to radiation, alcohol, drugs, nicotine, and many medications. Because enzymes are so fragile and because they face so many environmental and dietary factors conspiring to destroy them, we have to work hard to conserve our enzymes.

One way to replenish enzymes is by eating raw foods. Why? Because enzymes don't survive the cooking process; they begin to lose their activity at about 118°F. For those of us who live in cold climates, however, it's not always possible or even desirable to stick to a raw foods diet.

Still, no matter where we live, we can always eat some raw sprouts and blended salads—an excellent source of enzymes as well as an incomparable source of vitamins, minerals, and other beneficial elements. Sprouts are rich in phytochemicals—those plant-based nutrients so crucial to liver detox, cancer prevention, immunity, and defense against aging.

Enzyme-rich blended salads offer many of the same benefits as sprouts plus an additional bonus—chlorophyll. The use of fresh greens in blended salads provides a high supply of purifying chlorophyll and are also a great source of the vital detox mineral magnesium, involved with over 350 biochemical processes. (See all my blended salad recipes starting on page 208.)

It is interesting that the sprouting of seeds for their high enzyme value isn't a new idea at all. In fact, sprouting has been used for centuries. Sprouted mung beans have been a staple among the people of northern China, well known for their virility and youthful appearance—even when they've reached their hundredth birthday. In the eighteenth century, the British sprouted grains on ship to prevent their sailors from getting scurvy.

Seeds from grains, beans, and vegetables, especially lentils, alfalfa, mung beans, and radishes, lend themselves deliciously to sprouting. The sprouting process makes all of these plant foods much easier to digest because their starch is changed into sugar, making sprouts a terrifically high energy source that is easily absorbed and used by the body (see the Sprout-It-Yourself Method on page 207). Sprouts keep well in the fridge for about five days, after which they start to lose nutritional value.

So whether you sprout yourself (just remember to choose organic seeds) or pick up some fresh organic sprouts at your local health food store, you can easily incorporate the dynamic health value of fresh, enzyme-rich foods into your diet. Just throw some spicy radish sprouts into your salad, or top a stir-fry with mung bean sprouts. A dash of cumin or cayenne will bring out the sprouts' flavor and add some fire to your taste buds.

Nucleotides: Our Body's Genetic Building Blocks

FAST TRACK MAINSTAY: ONE CAN OF SARDINES OR 1 TO 2 TABLE-SPOONS OF YEAST FLAKES TWO TO FOUR TIMES A WEEK FOR ANTI-AGING NUCLEOTIDES

In the late 1970s, I came across a book titled *Dr. Frank's No-Aging Diet: Eat and Grow Younger.* I was fascinated by the possibilities the title suggested of eating and growing younger. On the front cover of the book it read, "The first diet book based on the scientific breakthrough of our age. Every cell in your body can be young again." Dr. Benjamin Frank wrote about the amazing rejuvenating properties of deoxyribonucleic acid (DNA) and ribonucleic acid (RNA). I was enthralled because DNA is the substance that contains the secret of life itself, whereas RNA is the messenger that carries these secrets to every single one of our cells. DNA and RNA are both nucleic acids, found in the nuclei of every living cell. And nucleotides are the building blocks for these extraordinary substances. Nucleotides are credited with helping our bodies repair themselves, creating new tissue, maintaining a strong immune system, and conducting many other important functions. That's probably why they're so highly concentrated in breast milk—and why they are now routinely added to infant formula. But we adults need them, too! Here's just a short list of what they do for us:[3]

- help neutralize toxins

- strengthen our immune system

- enhance the effects of antioxidants

- increase our ability to heal

- rev up our cellular metabolism and the production of cellular energy

- keep our skin supple and moist

- help restore hair growth and reverse the graying process

So Dr. Frank started to treat his patients with food and supplements containing high amounts of RNA. As he began replenishing nucleic acid in his patients' diets, he noticed that they began to look younger. Their aging process actually seemed to reverse, so that their wrinkles disappeared, their gray hair turned black, and their whole appearance became youthful and glowing. He had especially good re-

A NUCLEOTIDE-RICH SUPPLEMENT:
BLUE-GREEN ALGAE

If you'd like to sample another vegetarian source of nucleotides, I recommend E3Live, a form of blue-green algae officially known as *Aphanizomenon flos-aquae* (AFA). This food source is harvested from Upper Klamath Lake in southern Oregon, the only place in the world where large quantities of algae are available in the wild. Mindful of the reports that algae often harbors lethal doses of mercury, I reviewed product assays and made sure that no mercury was detected. I'm happy to recommend E3Live as a safe, organic food with no additives or pesticides, but with more than sixty-four vitamins and naturally chelated minerals that are 97 percent bioavailable to the body.

These algae are also an exceptional source of omega-3 fatty acids, carotenoids (antioxidants), and purifying chlorophyll. They contain phenylethylamine (PEA), an ingredient known as the "molecule of love," a potent mood-enhancer that combats depression, improves mental focus, and boosts energy. E3Live also contains phycocyanin, which makes the algae blue and is a

sults with skin conditions, reporting many cases of reversing acne in younger patients. He also frequently commented on dramatic new hair growth in his older patients once they started his diet.

Around the time I was first learning about nucleic acids, I was following a strict vegetarian diet, and so I made sure to get a daily dose of brewer's yeast to build up my vitamin B_{12}. (This was back in the days when nutritional yeast wasn't available, and brewer's yeast was the only yeast on the market.) To my surprise, my hair, which had been falling out after three months on my vegetarian diet, suddenly started to grow in thicker than ever. At the time, I attributed this new hair growth to the additional protein and B vitamins I was getting from the yeast. Today I realize that I was benefiting from the rejuvenating

powerful anti-inflammatory element. But this product's most unusual claim to fame is the polysaccharide it contains that stimulates the migration of "natural killer cells," those elements of your immune system that help kill off cancer and cells infected with viruses.

You can buy this product by phone or online (see "Resources"), and it's shipped to you frozen. For vegetarians or vegans relying on this as your primary protein source, you can take 2 tablespoons a day or more. If you're just looking for a living source of nucleotides, I recommend 1 or 1½ teaspoons a day.

TIP: Since the unfrozen shelf life of this product is only about seven days, you'll want to defrost the entire bottle in the fridge until you have about 3 tablespoons worth. Pour that into a smaller container and refreeze the rest of the bottle. Or you can defrost the whole bottle and pour the liquid into an ice cube tray. Freeze it again and store the cubes in an airtight container in your freezer. Drop a cube in water, and let it dissolve for an instant pick-me-up.

effects of the yeast's nucleic acids. This overlooked substance abounded in my old-fashioned brewer's yeast, and it's equally plentiful in today's more palatable and healthy nutritional yeast.

As you can see, nucleotides are not only crucial for detox but also for reversing the aging process. Sardines turn out to be one of the highest nucleic sources of all, along with other nucleic-acid-rich foods like seafood, radishes, asparagus, mushrooms, and onions. I recommend that you follow my nutritional recommendations for diet and detox, incorporating nutritional yeast or sardines as often as possible, but definitely two to four times a week.

Organic Foods: The Royal Road to Health and Weight Loss

Now that you've taken your body to the cleaners, you may be wondering where you go from here. As far as I'm concerned, the signs all point in one direction: *go organic*. You know by now that the most insidious factor making us Americans fat are those xenoestrogens we are exposed to every day, which make their way into our systems from pesticides, fertilizers, herbicides, antibiotics, preservatives, plastics, steroids, and growth hormones.

What's the point of getting all those toxins out of your system only to load yourself up again every time you sit down to dinner? All the detoxing in the world won't keep up with the load of chemicals you're consuming if you continue to eat conventionally farmed food.

Luckily, organic foods can be found in just about every supermarket these days. After all, organic was a $13 billion business in 2003, and it's growing every year. Even Wal-Mart has gotten into the act. And if you can't find what you need locally, you can always go online. So take the plunge! A commitment to buying organic food may be the single most powerful decision you can make to support your weight loss.

Organic: Is It Worth the Price?

Now by this point you may be thinking, "Sure, Ann Louise. I know organic foods are less toxic than conventionally farmed food. But they're also more expensive!" Believe me, I'm well aware of the problem. But as a nutritionist who works with literally thousands of dieters each year, I have to tell you what I know: The extra cost is absolutely justified by the benefits to your health, beauty, and ability to stay slim.

Organic foods are also sweeter, juicier, and so much more flavorful (just compare an organic tomato or carrot with a conventionally grown one and you'll see what I mean). And organic foods have far more nutrients than nonorganic foods. As a result, you fill up more quickly: Your taste buds as well as your stomach are satisfied and your body doesn't go begging for missing nutrients.

Consider the findings of researchers at Johns Hopkins University, who analyzed forty-one different studies conducted over a fifty-year period. They discovered that organic produce contained nearly 30 percent more vitamin C, more than 20 percent more iron, about 30 percent more magnesium, and 14 percent more phosphorus, as well as 15 percent fewer harmful nitrates than conventionally grown produce.[4] Clearly, you get what you pay for!

Organic farming also helps replenish the soil and is a mainstay for family farmers, the backbone of our nation. Staying on the organic track helps preserve our rivers, lakes, and streams from all those agricultural pollutants. It is a major step toward a healthier environment for us and for our children.

But in the end, I return to my original point. *If you want to lose weight, and keep it off, the only really effective way to do so is to eat organic.* So fill up your shopping cart with foods that bear the "USDA organic" label—and when you can't go organic, make the next-best choice. In the following sections, I'll talk you through your daily diet, helping you figure out how to "organize" your choices and how to choose healthy alternatives when organic is just not possible.

Powerful Proteins

FAST TRACK MAINSTAY: AT LEAST TWO SERVINGS (ABOUT THE SIZE OF THE PALM OF YOUR HAND) OF MEAT, CHICKEN OR FISH, PLUS TWO EGGS AND ONE TO TWO SERVINGS OF WHEY PER DAY FOR PROTEIN (VEGANS: EAT AT LEAST 2 TABLESPOONS OF BLUE-GREEN ALGAE, LIKE E3LIVE, PER DAY FOR PROTEIN.)

Red Meat

I'm a big fan of nostalgia. So I've got to tell you: Meat ain't what it used to be! Back in the days when cows roamed the meadows and ate grass instead of the grain they're fed now, they were clean and wholesome. Their meat was loaded with conjugated linoleic acid (CLA), the fat-burning fat that cows made from eating grass, a remarkable substance that helps the body replace fat with lean muscle.

CLA has also been shown to support the immune system, protect against heart disease, and inhibit the growth of some cancers. It may also help prevent and control adult-onset diabetes, along with bone loss, osteoporosis, and osteoarthritis.[5]

If the CLA in organic beef helps you lose weight, the xenoestrogens in nonorganic meats will fatten you up like a prize steer being prepared for market. That's not a figure of speech. Commercially raised cattle are given massive doses of growth hormone and fed on pesticide-laden grain. As a result, they take only one fifth as long as grass-fed organic cows to reach market weight. When we eat their nonorganic meat, we consume the estrogens they were given, which both raises our weight and may expose us to increased risk of breast cancer.[6]

The European Union is so concerned about these steroids that they've banned them. So have U.S. organic producers. And what's the result? The steak from organic grass-fed cattle has only about half the fat of grain-fed sirloin, not to mention more CLA and about four times more omega-3 fat-burning fatty acids. Organic meat costs more because the cows take five times longer to bring to market, but I hope you're beginning to see why the price is worth it.[7]

There's one more health hazard lurking in nonorganic beef—

antibiotics. Did you know that some 70 percent of all the antibiotics used in the United States are given to healthy livestock? These medications creep into our systems, killing off the friendly bacteria that we need, and creating antibiotic-resistant strains of bacteria. That's why the World Health Organization (WHO) has recommended banning antibiotics in animal feed and why the European Union is phasing out their use. I recommend you do the same, by buying meat labeled "no antibiotics administered" or "raised without antibiotics."[8]

For those of you consuming whey, make sure it's the product of hormone-free cows. You can count on Fat Flush Whey to be hormone-free.

Now that you know what's at stake (no pun intended), here are some tips for how to fill your diet with tasty, clean, organic red meat:

- Buy beef that is labeled "grass-fed," "organic," and "no antibiotics administered" or "raised without antibiotics."

- For those times you absolutely can't get grass-fed beef, add more essential oils to your diet, such as omega-3-rich flaxseed soil and fish oil. Grass-fed beef is far higher in omega-3 fats, so if you're eating grain-fed meat, you need to get your omega-3s in another way. Make sure any fish oil supplement you take is derived from fish-body oils, not fish-liver oils, and is molecularly distilled to remove mercury, PCBs, heavy metals, and other contaminants.

- Consider substituting wild game (only 3.9 percent fat) for beef and pork (up to 35 percent fat). Try elk, venison, yak, and even buffalo or bison for an iron-rich, low-fat protein source. Game is also higher in omega-3s and CLA than grain-fed cattle, and contains fewer pesticides.

- Consider substituting lamb for beef. Like game, lambs are cleaner animals than fully grown cows, because their meat contains fewer pesticides.

- Pass on the pork. My good friend Dr. Hal Huggins has confirmed something I've always believed—that "the other white meat" is simply not good for humans. That's because pigs have no means of sweating except through their hooves, so pigs are more likely to retain toxins than other animals. If you're a pork fan, may I suggest the following experiment? Give it up for thirty days, and then try a serving. You may be surprised at how difficult you find it to digest and how many toxic symptoms you develop when your system has a chance to clear.

Poultry and Eggs

Although for a while, heart-conscious dieters were being told to eat less red meat and more poultry, commercially grown chickens may be even worse for your health than grain-fed cattle. Studies have shown that some 30 percent of commercially raised chickens suffer from *Salmonella* contamination, whereas more than 60 percent have *Campylobacter,* a bacteria found in fecal material.

And, just like cows, our commercially raised poultry is loaded with antibiotics—up to 10.5 million pounds a year, according to the Union of Concerned Scientists.[9]

The solution? Buy organic or kosher. Don't be fooled by the label "free range," either. That only means that the bird was allowed out into a yard for a few minutes a day. You want to look for labels reading "certified organic" and "USDA organic" to ensure that the birds were raised without antibiotics. "Free farmed" and "Food Alliance" will also do the trick. And "pasture-raised" means the chicken or turkey was actually allowed to roam about in a more natural setting.

And when it comes to eggs, it's organic eggs all the way. Look for eggs enriched with omega-3, which have over 400 percent more essential fatty acids (EFAs) than regular eggs.

Fish

Even the American Heart Association (AHA) recommends eating fish twice a week to get the benefits of omega-3 fats. But the AHA shares my concern about the mercury and PCBs turning up in our fishy friends. In fact, both the FDA and the EPA have warned children and pregnant women to avoid or limit their intake of certain types of fish, so as not to consume the mercury, PCBs, and dioxins that pollute our oceans, lakes, and streams. They—and you—should take particular care to avoid shark, swordfish, king mackerel, and tilefish.

One of the major concerns about fish is their contamination with mercury, which is a potent and deadly neurotoxin that may be linked to multiple sclerosis, Alzheimer's disease, Hodgkin's disease, chronic fatigue syndrome, and virtually all autoimmune disorders, as well as cardiovascular and reproductive system diseases. When mercury meets the bacteria that live in fresh and salt water, it becomes methyl mercury, an even deadlier form of the heavy metal. It works its way into the algae growing in fresh and salt water. Little fish eat the algae, big fish eat the little fish, and the methyl mercury piles up.

I wish I could just tell you to buy organic fish, but I can't. That's because the U.S. Department of Agriculture (USDA) has never certified standards for organic fish, mainly because there is no organic food available to feed farmed fish. It's kind of a vicious circle: Farmed fish eat fish meal, but then you'd need organic fish to make the meal. In fact, farmed fish are eating fairly dangerous food, as studies have found higher levels of PCBs in farmed fish than in their wild counterparts.[10]

A 2003 study from the Environmental Working Group found that farmed salmon grown in the United States have up to sixteen times the PCBs found in wild salmon. Farmed salmon are even higher in PCBs than beef (four times), let along other seafood (about three and a half times).[11]

The solution? Focus on the healthier, smaller types of fish and avoid the ones that are piling up the mercury. I also urge you to choose those species that are harvested in sustainable ways, to show respect for our oceans' bounty. Use "Fish Picks" to help you sort through the choices.

FISH PICKS

FISH TO CHOOSE: Alaskan pollock, bluefish, catfish (farmed), canned mackerel, cod caught with hook and line, croaker, flounder (summer), mahi-mahi, Pacific halibut, sablefish, striped bass, tilapia, trout (farmed), salmon (wild Pacific and Alaskan)

SHELLFISH TO CHOOSE: Atlantic northern pink shrimp, blue crab (not from Chesapeake Bay), crawfish, farmed clams, farmed scallops, trap-caught spot prawns

FISH TO LOSE: Atlantic cod, Atlantic halibut, Atlantic salmon, grouper, haddock, orange roughy, Pacific rockfish, Patagonian toothfish (also known as Chilean sea bass), red snapper, swordfish, canned and fresh tuna

SHELLFISH TO LOSE: Chesapeake Bay blue crab, dredged clams, dredged scallops, lobster, shrimp[12]

ATLANTIC VS. ALASKA: HOW TO CHOOSE?

Clearly, you should avoid farmed salmon and focus on the wild variety. But you may have to put a bit of effort into this choice: more than 70 percent of the fresh salmon eaten in the United States is farmed. As of 2004, distributors have to label their salmon's country of origin, and whether the salmon is wild or farmed. For those of you who eat in restaurants, salmon labeled "Atlantic" is farmed, so look for the label that says "Alaska." Whether canned or fresh, Alaskan wild salmon beats Atlantic farmed salmon every time.[13]

Delicious Dairy

FAST TRACK MAINSTAY: ONE TO TWO SERVINGS OF DAIRY (I/2 CUP RICOTTA OR COTTAGE CHEESE, I CUP YOGURT, OR I OUNCE CHEESE) PER DAY (OPTIONAL)

Everything you've read about beef cattle applies to commercially raised dairy cows as well. Like their beefy cousins, dairy cattle are raised in crowded, miserable conditions, dosed with huge helpings of antibiotics to prevent the spread of disease, and spurred to unnatural rates of milk production with such hormones as recombinant bovine growth hormone (rBGH). These additives pass right into the cows' milk, cheese, and yogurt, with the familiar disastrous results for our health and weight.

Recombinant bovine growth hormone is a particularly dangerous addition to our milk products. This product of the Monsanto Corporation is a genetically engineered means of speeding up a cow's metabolism, causing it to release up to 25 percent more milk—and also, perhaps to pass on a substance to us milk drinkers that has been associated with breast, colon, and prostate cancer. Cows dosed with rBGH are also more vulnerable to disease, which means they also tend to get more antibiotics. And both rBGH and antibiotics disrupt *our* hormones, inducing estrogen dominance, a host of symptoms, and weight gain.[14]

So look for milk and dairy products that are marked "rBGH-free" or labeled "no growth hormones." And look for products made from goat's and sheep's milk, since these two mammals are not (yet) fed any form of rBGH.

Making Healthy Choices with Fruits and Veggies

FAST TRACK MAINSTAY: TWO SERVINGS PER DAY OF FRUIT

FAST TRACK MAINSTAY: FIVE SERVINGS (ABOUT THE SIZE OF A FULL COFFEE MUG) PER DAY OF VEGETABLES

Recently, I was on an out-of-town business trip, and my host wanted to take me to lunch in a nice restaurant. The special salad of the day

CHEESE PICKS

CHEESES TO CHOOSE: raw milk Swiss or Cheddar, goat's milk cheese or chèvre (Montrachet, banon, and Bûcheron), sheep's milk cheese like green feta or French Roquefort Buffalo mozzarella; any cheese from Canada, Australia, New Zealand, and the European Union, all of which have banned growth hormone.

CHEESES TO LOSE: All other American-made cheese from cow's milk, including Cheddar, Swiss, and Jack.

I CAN'T BELIEVE IT'S GRASS-FED BUTTER!

When it comes to weight loss, butter and cream can be either your best friends or your worst enemies. Because butter and cream are fats, they're a storehouse for pesticides and antibiotics if they're made from commercially farmed, grain-fed animals. When these products are made from grass-fed and organically raised animals, however, they are an excellent source of fat-burning conjugated linoleic acid (CLA). So if you can find butter and cream made from grass-fed, organically raised cows, enjoy them to your heart's content. But stay away from all nonorganic butter and cream.

was made from baby spinach, which, I admit, sounded delicious. But knowing what I knew about pesticides and chemical fertilizers, I just could not bring myself to eat nonorganic spinach, which is one of the most heavily sprayed vegetables grown in this country. Instead of the tender green leaves, glistening under their dressing, all I could picture was the droplets of the forty pesticides found on spinach during government tests.[15] Regretfully, I asked the waiter if the salad could be prepared with romaine lettuce instead.

My lunchtime host looked on in amazement. "I thought I was being healthy by eating five vegetables and two fruits a day," he said. "Are you telling me that's not enough?"

No, I replied with regret. It wasn't. Every time you throw a handful of nonorganic strawberries into your morning smoothie, you're dosing yourself with captan, a fungicide that's been linked to cancer; birth defects; and damage to the immune, nervous, and reproductive systems. Each time you bite into a fresh, fiber-rich nonorganic apple, you're exposing yourself to diphenylamine, which in laboratory studies was shown to cause damage to the brain and nervous system. And whenever you crunch on a stick of celery—even as part of your Three-Day Sequel—you're getting a serving of permethrin, chlorothalonil, and acephate along with your fiber; these pesticides have been linked to cancer.[16] So your efforts to create a healthy, nutritious, and slenderizing diet will never "bear fruit" if you don't avoid the most toxic nonorganic produce. In the ideal world, I'd simply tell you that every piece of fruit you buy, every single vegetable, every plant food of any kind, must absolutely be organic. That's still the best rule of thumb.

So remember: *When you can, buy organic. When you can't, make the healthiest choices you can.* At least you can stay away from the Top 10 Toxic Fruits—strawberries, cherries, apples, Mexican cantaloupe, apricots, blackberries, pears, raspberries, and fresh peaches (canned are not so bad). You should also stay away from the most toxic vegetables—nonorganic spinach, hot and sweet peppers, celery, and potatoes. When you can't buy organic, buy less-toxic substitutes: blueberries instead of strawberries; chard instead of spinach; bananas instead of apples. See "Veggie Picks" to help you sort through the choices.

Starches

FAST TRACK MAINSTAY: UP TO 4 DAILY SERVINGS PER DAY OF CEREALS, GRAINS, BREADS, OR LEGUMES

If you enjoy cereals, grains, and legumes, try to choose the USDA organic label. Brands like Erewhon, Arrowhead Mills, and Seeds of Change are safe bets. French Meadow Bakery has an entire line of or-

VEGGIE PICKS

High-pesticide fruits and veggies

BUY ORGANIC IF POSSIBLE, OR SUBSTITUTE WITH ANOTHER CHOICE:[17]

apples, apricots, artichokes, cantaloupe from Mexico, celery, cherries from the United States, grapes from Chile, peaches, pears, potatoes, raspberries, spinach, strawberries

Lower in pesticides

WHEN YOU CAN'T BUY ORGANIC, CHOOSE THESE:

asparagus, avocados, bananas, blackberries, blueberries, broccoli, Brussels sprouts, cabbage, cantaloupe from the United States (in season from May to December), carrots, cauliflower, chard, corn, eggplant, grapefruit, grapes from the United States (in season from May to December), kiwi, lettuce (Romaine), okra, onions, peaches (canned), peas, radishes, tangerines, tomatoes, watermelon

ganic breads (HealthSeed Spelt, Men's Bread, Woman's Bread) and tortillas (including their Fat Flush Tortilla which is made from sprouted organic grains).

The Essential and Healing Fats

FAST TRACK MAINSTAY: UP TO 2 TABLESPOONS PER DAY OF OILS, NUTS, AND SEEDS

Fats and oils can be one of the healthiest substances in your diet—but only if they're organic. The oils in commercially grown seeds and nuts can be a storehouse of fattening pesticides—we're not the only life forms to store toxins in fat, so do look for the organic label. You can find organic flaxseed oil and olive oil in most health food stores and you can find organic olive oil and coconut oil on supermarket shelves. Organic peanut butter, almond butter, and sesame seed butter are also easily available, as are organic almonds, walnuts, macadamia nuts, Brazil nuts, hickory nuts, peanuts, sunflower seeds, and sesame seeds. I like Health from the Sun, Omega, and Spectrum brands for healthy salad oil, and Arrowhead Mills and Natural Value for the tastiest nut butters.

More Detox Options

Throughout this book, we've talked about detox through diet, which I have advocated for many years and continue to believe must be the centerpiece of any weight-loss plan in our toxic world. But there are numerous nonchemical detox approaches that I think make a healthy supplement to the Fast Track. Besides being healthy and conducive to weight loss, they also feel terrific!

- *Dry saunas.* Here you achieve detox by sweating toxins out through the skin. When you remember that the skin is your largest external organ, it's not a bad idea to take advantage of its size to help eliminate heavy metals and other toxins, particularly since that helps relieve some of the stress on the liver and kidneys. Don't overdo it, however. Start with a five- or ten-minute sauna at 135°F. Gradually work your way up to a forty-five-minute sauna; and then, after a month or so, increase the temperature to 145°F. You may have difficulty finding a sauna that cool, because many spas and gyms feature saunas with temperatures as high as 195°F, which I do *not* recommend—the stress on your system outweighs any benefits you might derive from the detox. But you may be able to rent space in the sauna at a local hotel (where you will have an easier time controlling the temperature) or even to buy your own infrared sauna.[18]

- *Parcells hot baths.* I owe these formulas to my mentor, Dr. Hazel Parcells, a pioneer in alternative medicine. I rely on them myself, and I'm delighted to pass them on to you. But don't take more than one bath a day—and don't mix baths!

FORMULA 1: TO HELP DETOX FROM RADIATION EXPOSURE DURING AIR TRAVEL, DENTAL EXAM, MAMMOGRAM, RADIATION THERAPY, OR PROXIMITY TO A NUCLEAR PLANT:

- Run a tub to the hottest temperature you can manage. Dissolve 1 pound of salt and 1 pound of baking soda in the water, and begin to soak.

- Sip a glass of warm water mixed with 1/2 teaspoon of salt and 1/2 teaspoon of baking soda.

- Get out of the bath when the water is cool. Don't shower for at least four hours.

FORMULA 2: TO HELP DETOX FROM METAL POISONING INDUCED BY ALUMINUM COOKWARE, YOUR SILVER AMALGAMS, OR ANTACIDS; FROM THE CARBON MONOXIDE INHALED IN HEAVY TRAFFIC; OR FROM PESTICIDE EXPOSURE:

- Run a tub to the hottest temperature you can manage. Pour 1 cup of Clorox bleach into the water—but no more!—and begin to soak.

- Get out of the bath when the water is cool. Don't shower for at least four hours.

FORMULA 3: TO HELP DETOX FROM IRRADIATED FOOD AND FOOD-BORNE BACTERIA, INCLUDING *E. COLI* AND *SALMONELLA*:

- Run a tub to the hottest temperature you can manage. Pour in 2 pounds of baking soda.

- Sip a glass of warm water mixed with 1/2 teaspoon of baking soda.

- Get out of the bath when the water is cool. Don't shower for at least four hours.

FORMULA 4: TO HELP BUILD IMMUNITY BY RAISING YOUR BODY'S ACIDITY, WHICH MAKES YOU LESS HOSPITABLE "TERRAIN" FOR BACTERIA AND VIRUSES; GOOD FOR PREVENTING ILLNESSES:

- Run a tub to the hottest temperature you can manage. Pour in 2 cups of organic apple cider vinegar.

- Sip a glass of warm water mixed with 1 tablespoon organic apple cider vinegar.

- Get out of the bath when the water is cool. Don't shower for at least four hours.[19]

Three Paths to Health and Weight Loss: Which Will You Choose?

Now that you've got a sense of how terrific detox feels, and how important it is for weight loss, it's time to decide where you'll go from here. I've given you all the tools I can to help you craft your own eating plan, so if you've already got a vision for how you want to take the Fast Track to the next level, more power to you!

But just in case you'd like a bit more guidance, I've come up with three approaches to diet and detox—a range of choices that offer something to every dieter out there. Perhaps, like Jewelle, you're committed to going organic all the way. In that case, Path A, the Fastest Track, is tailor-made for you, an approach that enables you to stay slim, trim, and detoxed while making healthy, organic choices as often as you can. Maybe, like Mercedes, you're looking for an approach to eating that will allow you a certain amount of indulgence, a chance to sample wine, desserts, and other "forbidden" foods at least occasionally, while still staying in shape. Then you'll probably want to explore Path B, the Cheater's Diet, which makes room for a wider variety of choices while encouraging you to stay within healthy boundaries. And if, like Connor, you choose to stay on the Fat Flush Plan, Path C, the Fat Flush Mix and Match, will show you how to integrate fasting into your Fat Flush program.

No matter which way you choose, you should keep the Fast Track Mainstays in mind. They are your basic building blocks for a healthy diet, the primary checklist you should use to make sure you're getting all nutrients you need to support your liver, colon, and digestive system. What I like about this approach is that it gives you a basic minimum to shoot for, a nutritional "floor" that will support you even during the most stressful and confusing times. And who knows? Once you've started eating the Fast Track way, you may find yourself making new choices in your diet, lifestyle, and life choices. The sky's the limit!

Path A: The Fastest Track

Congratulations! By choosing Path A, you're agreeing to make detox dieting a way of life and creating a plan you can live with. You are committed to choosing organic and wholesome foods of the highest quality as an integral part of your daily eating, both because they offer superior taste and higher nutritional content and because they are good for the planet. You're raising your awareness about the toxic sea of chemicals in which we live, and you're doing your best to reduce your own body's chemical burden by making lifestyle changes that are limiting your exposure to toxins in food, air, water, cooking utensils, personal-care products, and your home. As an added bonus, you'll never have trouble keeping weight off or maintaining your natural beauty!

A Closer Look at Path A

Buy as Close to 100 Percent Organic as Your Budget or Geographical Location Will Allow

Earlier in this chapter, you learned that the Top 10 Toxic (pesticide-ridden) Fruits are strawberries, cherries, apples, Mexican cantaloupe, apricots, blackberries, pears, raspberries, grapes from Chile, and peaches. So you need to buy only organic versions of these fruits.

Can't always find these organic and fresh? No problem. Companies like Cascadian Farms provide frozen organic fruits like strawberries, cherries, blackberries, raspberries, and peaches all year round. To me, these frozen organic fruits are actually a much better buy than the fresh variety because they are uniformly sweet and flavorful. Fresh berries, by the time they reach the market, are often overripe and spoiled from handling. Those at the bottom of the basket are sometimes crushed and inedible. Mold forms almost instantly on a crushed berry. You don't have any of those problems with frozen fruit.

Luckily, most of the Liver-Loving veggies that you will be eating each day are among the least contaminated plant foods. So you can safely enjoy broccoli, Brussels sprouts, cauliflower, artichokes, asparagus, leafy greens (except for spinach), and radishes.

When it comes to other kinds of vegetables, though, it's "eater beware." Spinach, hot and sweet peppers, celery, and potatoes are the Top 4 Toxic Veggies. So if you're in a restaurant, try to substitute sweet potatoes for regular potatoes, and tell the waiter to leave out all the peppers and celery from your salad. And bring on the garlic—it's always good for you!

You can definitely afford to be picky when it comes to protein. To avoid all those hormones and antibiotics:

- Get your protein from organic, free-range, and grass-fed sources as much as possible (see "Resources" for where to purchase these proteins).

- Remember to avoid chickens that do drugs! Organic, free-range poultry (both chicken and turkey) is available nationwide in both health food stores and in supermarkets.

- Omega-3-enriched eggs from egg producers like Eggland's Best and Pilgrim's Pride EggsPlus not only taste better but have the brightest and cleanest-tasting yolks you have ever seen.

- Choose either organic dairy, European dairy, or dairy made from sheep's milk and goat's milk.

- Stay away from farmed fish. See "Fish Picks" on page 158.

Use the Healthiest Food Combinations

Each food category (protein, fruit, starch, etc.) requires a different type of enzyme for proper digestion. At the risk of sounding simplistic, the healthiest food combinations are those in which the enzymes used to

PATH A: THE FASTEST TRACK

- Eat all the Fast Track Mainstays.

- Avoid all Detox Detractors.

- Undertake the Fast Track One-Day Detox Diet at least once a month and as often as bimonthly. Because you are consistently eating Liver-Loving and Colon-Caring Foods and avoiding all Detox Detractors, you are in tip-top shape to detox.

- Buy as close to 100 percent organic as your budget or geographical location will allow.

- *Use the healthiest food combinations and avoid the least healthy combinations.*

Combinations to choose:

> Protein and green vegetables
>
> Starch and vegetables
>
> Melons eaten alone
>
> Other fruits eaten at the beginning of a meal or between meals (except fruit with yogurt)
>
> Eggs, which are neutral and can be enjoyed in most combinations

Combinations to lose:

> Flesh proteins (beef, veal, lamb, chicken, or fish) and gluten-rich grain starches (wheat, rye, oats and barley, which you shouldn't be eating too much of anyway)
>
> Vegetables and fruit
>
> Milk and meat

- *Take the following basic dietary supplements:*

> A daily female or male multiple vitamin and mineral supplement

Antioxidant supplements (vitamin C, 2 to 5 grams daily, vitamin E, 400 to 1200 International Units daily; Oxy-Key, 2 to 4 tablets, one to three times daily)

Omega-3 fish oil supplements (with EPA and DHA), 1 to 3 grams daily (made from molecularly distilled fish-body oils free of mercury, PCBs, heavy metals, and other contaminants)

GLA, 360 milligrams daily

HCl and pepsin with ox bile, 1 to 3 tablets, three times daily with meals

Extra carb-controlling, fat-metabolizing, and liver-supporting nutrients, such as the Weight Loss Formula (see page 172)

- *Avoid the use of microwave ovens for cooking.*
- *Avoid plastics and aluminum when preparing or storing foods.*
- *Avoid cosmetics with the following ingredients:*

Imidazolidinyl urea and diazolidinyl urea (germall II and germall 115)

Methyl and propyl and butyl and ethyl paraben

Petrolatum

Propylene glycol

PVP/VA copolymer

Sodium lauryl sulfate

Stearalkonium chloride

Synthetic colors (labeled FD&C or D&C, followed by a color and a number)

Synthetic fragrances (labeled fragrance in the ingredients list)

Triethanolamine

digest various food groups do not compete for the gut's attention, avoiding the putrefaction that comes with undigested food. Because digestion is so central to proper absorption and assimilation of nutrients, it's worth your while to arrange your meals in such a way that the enzymes used to digest each food group are kept separated from one another.

Take the Most Fortifying Supplements for Maintaining the Fastest Track Health

A Daily Female or Male Multiple Vitamin and Mineral Supplement

Premenopausal women should look for an all-in-one daily multivitamin designed to meet a woman's special needs that is also safe for pregnant (just in case) and breast-feeding women. You want a multi that is copper free, since excessive levels of copper have been associated with estrogen dominance, which is linked in turn to water retention and weight gain. You should also look for a supplement that contains two times more magnesium than calcium to optimize calcium absorption for strong bones and relaxed muscles. Menopausal and postmenopausal women should take the multivitamin that I recommend for men (see "Resources").

Men, you need a multiple that is specifically designed with key vitamins and minerals that are essential for the male body and that is also iron free. A high level of iron in the bloodstream is considered a major risk factor for heart disease, still the number one degenerative disease in the United States, and for arthritis and other disorders. Since men aren't losing blood every month, they have to be careful about not taking in too much iron (see "Resources").

Antioxidant Supplements: Vitamin C (2 to 5 grams daily), Vitamin E (400 to 1200 IU daily), Oxi-Key (2 to 4 tablets, one to three times daily)

You already know how crucial antioxidants are to both the Phase 1 and Phase 2 liver detox pathways and to maintaining your health in general to fight oxidative stress. Oxy-Key is a particularly powerful supplement that I take myself, and is based on a clinically tested anti-oxidant. One tablet contains the following ingredients:

Catalase, 14,000 units

Superoxide dismutase, 6,000 units

Glutathione, 25 millgrams

N-acetyl cysteine, 12 milligrams

L-Cysteine, 15 milligrams

Vitamin B$_2$ (riboflavin), 4 milligrams

Vitamin E (natural), 14 International Units

Thioproline, 1,200 micrograms

Omega-3—Fish Oil Supplements with EPA and DHA (1 to 3 grams daily)

The omega-3 essential fatty acids enhance glucose regulation and help reverse insulin resistance, both of which actions ultimately support weight control. EPA (eicosapentanoic acid) and DHA (docosahexanoic acid) are essential fatty acids that are also anti-inflammatory agents. They play a key role in cardiovascular, brain, joint, and immune system health.

Omega-6—GLA Supplements from Black Currant Seed Oil (360 milligrams daily)

Omega-6, an essential fatty acid, is a natural weight-loss aid that triggers the metabolism of brown adipose tissue (BAT) and acts as a natural diuretic by balancing the body's sodium–potassium pump.

HCl and Pepsin with Ox Bile (1 to 3 tablets, three times daily with meals)

Hydrochloric acid is essential for the digestion of protein and acid-based minerals such as calcium, magnesium, and iron. As we saw in chapter 3, many of us suffer from low levels of stomach acid and can benefit from supplemental help. Take the Hydrochloride Challenge (page 50) to find out whether you need to take HCl and, if so, exactly how much you may personally need to support your own digestive needs.

Extra Carb-Controlling, Fat-Metabolizing, and Liver-Supporting Nutrients (the Weight Loss Formula)

The Weight Loss Formula, which is the centerpiece of the Fat Flush Kit, includes various B vitamins as well as chromium to help calm carbohydrate cravings. It also contains l-carnitine, methionine, inositol, and lipase to assist in digestion and metabolism of carbs and fats. Finally, the formula contains special herbal support for the liver. Here's the complete list of ingredients (amounts are for three capsules):

Vitamin B_3 (niacin), 15 milligrams

Vitamin B_6 (pyridoxine hydrochloride), 20 milligrams

Vitamin C (ascorbic acid), 100 milligrams

Choline (bitartrate), 335 milligrams

Inositol, 335 milligrams

Chromium (Chromate brand polynicotinate), 400 micrograms

l-Lysine hydrochloride, 100 milligrams

Methionine, 100 milligrams

l-Carnitine (tartrate), 500 milligrams

Lecithin, 100 milligrams

Lipase plant enzyme (30,000 units/gram; from *Aspergillus, oryzae*), 200 milligrams

Lipotropic Herbal Blend (whole turmeric, dandelion root, milk thistle, Oregon grape root), 200 milligrams

---

THE FAST DETOX DIET KIT

For those of you on the go, you can rely on the Fast Detox Diet Kit as your dietary insurance for life. The kit contains a month's supply of:

1. Super-GI Cleanse: a source of colon-cleansing fiber, plus herbs that target your eliminating organs

2. Liver-Lovin' Formula: designed to support your liver

3. Flora-Key: a powdered source of probiotics for complete gastrointestinal health.

To order, call 800-888-4353, or see my Web site (www.fast trackdetox.com).

Avoid the Use of Microwave Ovens for Cooking

Microwaves are a form of electromagnetic energy, like radio waves or light waves. Although they've become increasingly popular as a way of reheating or even cooking food, I've never been comfortable with them, and neither have many of my colleagues. In his recently published *Politically Incorrect Nutrition*, Michael Barbee reports on U.S. researcher William Kopp, who in the 1970s examined research conducted by Soviet scientists into what was then a new technology. Kopp's review of the Soviet research turned up some interesting—and shocking—facts about food cooked with microwaves, which included

- carcinogens that developed in some meats, milk, and cereal grains

- a rise in stomach and intestinal cancers among those who ate microwaved foods

- dysfunctions in the digestive and lymphatic systems of those who ate microwaved foods

- the formation of free radicals

- a decline in the bioavailability of many nutrients

- destabilized proteins

Moreover, Kopp found, all the foods that the Soviets had studied were damaged in some way.

Kopp's findings haven't been corroborated in this country, and many unanswered questions about this popular technology remain. But I, for one, think it's better to be safe than sorry. If you can find another way to cook or reheat your food, I suggest you rely on the old-fashioned stove or even your toaster oven and leave microwaves to the phone company. Otherwise, you may be adding a dose of carcinogens to your diet every time you "nuke" a meal.[19]

Avoid Plastics and Aluminum when Preparing or Storing Foods

Okay, this may be the worst news I've ever had to give you: *Don't use cling wrap.* I know it's convenient—and ubiquitous. When I shop in my local supermarket, it seems as though virtually every piece of produce, cheese, and meat is wrapped in it. But that particular type of soft plastic will only encourage toxins to migrate from the plastic right into your food.

Generally, you should avoid plastics as much as possible, storing food in glass or ceramic containers. Aluminum-proof your kitchen: Get rid of any aluminum cookware you still have hanging around the house and use only stainless steel or glass to prepare your food. Check all steamers, measuring cups, bread pans, and cookie sheets, and make sure you replace them with items made from Pyrex, stainless steel, or dairy tin. I also recommend replacing any baking powders with alu-

minum (as well as deodorants or antiperspirants) to reduce your overall exposure to aluminum buildup. Aluminum tends to accumulate,
bit by bit, in your organs, muscles, and tissues, with a host of toxic results.

I recommend heavy stainless-steel waterless cookware, which
cooks food in its own juices in a vacuum seal. Although it's more expensive than regular stainless, the waterless type of pot or pan will help
keep the vitamins and minerals in your food, where they belong.
Enamel-covered Le Creuset is also an excellent choice, as is Corning-
Ware.

For baking, rely on heavy-duty tin or black steel. Use only glass
or stainless steel bowls, especially for food storage. And instead of aluminum foil for cooking and reheating, use parchment paper. Because
paper-wrapped food cooks in its own juices, both nutrients and flavor remain within the food. You can buy it in most grocery stores and
health food stores.

Avoid cosmetics with the following ingredients:

- **Imidazolidinyl urea and diazonlidinyl urea (germall II and germall 115):** these ingredients are a primary cause of contact dermatitis.

- **Methyl and propyl and butyl and ethyl paraben:** the parabens
  tend to induce allergic reactions and skin rashes.

- **Petrolatum:** you put yourself at risk of a host of symptoms with
  this mineral oil and jelly, including photosensitivity, dry skin, and
  chapping.

- **Propylene glycol:** there is a natural form of this substance, but
  many cosmetics use a synthetic form that is the equivalent of
  antifreeze and can cause allergic and toxic reactions.

- **PVP/VA copolymer:** this petroleum-derived chemical—used in
  hair sprays, wave sets, and cosmetics—can contribute to foreign
  bodies accumulating in the lungs of sensitive people.

- **Sodium lauryl sulfate:** a common ingredient in shampoos, sodium lauryl sulfate can cause eye irritations, skin rashes, hair loss, a dandruff-like scalp buildup, and allergic reactions.

- **Stearalkonium chloride:** used in hair conditioners and creams, this substance can provoke allergic reactions.

- **Synthetic colors (labeled "FD&C" or "D&C," followed by a color and a number):** these synthetic color-causing chemicals may be carcinogenic.

- **Synthetic fragrances (labeled "fragrance" in the ingredients list):** fragrances may be composed of more than 200 ingredients. Often, they induce headaches, dizziness, rashes, coughing, vomiting, skin irritation, and hyperpigmentation (your skin turning an intense color).

- **Triethanolamine:** This substance, TEA for short, can cause allergic reactions, dry hair, and dry skin.

As we've seen, your skin is your largest detox organ, capable of expelling toxins via perspiration released through the pores. By the same token, toxins applied *to* your skin likewise enter into your system. So to the extent you can, avoid petrochemical-based cosmetics, including mineral oil, petrolatum, synthetic colors, and synthetic fragrances.

Path B: The Cheater's Diet

Cheating can be okay if you give yourself some insurance. By eating organic when you can and making healthy choices when you can't, you're doing a great deal to keep toxins out of your body. By loading yourself up with fruits, veggies, healthy fats, and the other elements of the Fast Track Mainstays, you're ensuring that you get the nutrients you need. And by fasting periodically, you're taking off the extra pounds that "cheating" might put on, as well as cleansing your system of all the toxins you ingest by eating nonorganic food. Maybe someday you'll be ready to try out Path A—but for now, this is the right choice for you.

PATH B: THE CHEATER'S DIET

- Eat all the Fast Track Mainstays.

- Allow yourself one Detox Detractor per week, but take a special formula designed to support your adrenal glands, your body's stress glands.

- Undertake the Fast Track One-Day Detox Diet anywhere from once a month to once every two months. Be sure to avoid all Detox Detractors during the Seven-Day Prequel and during the Three-Day Sequel. Your one-day fast will help you take off any extra pounds you put on while helping to rid your body of toxins.

- Buy at least 50 percent organic, and make healthy choices according to the lists given in this chapter.

- Every day, take the supplements from the Fast Detox Diet Kit (page 173).

- Take an antiyeast formula, such as the homeopathic Y-C Cleanse, Pau D'Arco tea, or oil of oregano to help fight your sugar cravings.

A Closer Look at Path B

Eat All the Fast Track Mainstays

For you, it's extra-important to load up on enzyme-rich sprouts and the nucleotide-rich foods I've recommended: sardines, asparagus, mushrooms, radishes, and beets. And don't forget your daily serving of probiotic sauerkraut or yogurt, to keep those friendly bacteria flourishing.

*Allow Yourself One Detox Detractor Per Week, but
Take a Nutrient-Rich Formula Designed to Support
Your Adrenal Glands*

In my experience, sugar and caffeine cravings aren't a matter of willpower. They're classic symptoms of a person who's suffering from adrenal burnout. Your adrenal glands are what manufacture the stress hormones you need to meet a particularly challenging situation, whether meeting a tight deadline for work or coping with the death of a loved one. Chronic stress weakens the adrenal glands and leads to "burnout"—the exhaustion of these vital body parts and their inability to produce enough stress hormones to help you stay energized and focused. Lethargy, listlessness, and fatigue are the results—and caffeine or sugar can seem like a solution.

So nourish your poor, starved adrenals with something more helpful than either sugar or caffeine, which, as you know, can create as many crashes and lows as they produce rushes and highs. To balance your body chemistry, take a dietary supplement that provides all the key vitamins, minerals, glandular tissues, and amino acids your body needs when under stress.

You might want to try The Adrenal Formula (see "Resources"). One tablet contains the following: Vitamin A (palmitate), 5,000 International Units; vitamin C (ascorbic acid), 175 milligrams; vitamin B_5 (di-calcium pantothenate), 25 milligrams; vitamin B_6 (pyroxidine hydrochloride), 15 milligrams; zinc (citrate), 5 milligrams; tyrosine, 175 milligrams; raw bovine adrenal (freeze-dried), 200 milligrams; Raw Bovine Adrenal cortex (freeze dried), 15 milligrams; raw bovine spleen, 100 milligrams; and raw bovine liver, 25 milligrams.

*Buy at Least 50 Percent Organic, and Make Healthy
Choices According to the Lists Given in This Chapter*

You'd be surprised at how much of a difference it makes to switch to organic foods—even partway. If you liked the purified, energized, and wholesome feeling you got from your One-Day Detox Diet, keep that detox sensation alive by keeping your diet as organic as possible and avoiding the worst offenders. In fruits, stay away from nonorganic strawberries, cherries, apples, Mexican cantaloupe, apricots, blackberries, pears, raspberries, grapes from Chile, and peaches; in veggies, avoid celery, hot and sweet peppers, spinach, and potatoes. And remember, frozen foods are a terrific and affordable organic alternative (see "Resources").

Take an Antiyeast Formula, Such as the Homeopathic Y-C Cleanse, Pau D'Arco Tea, or Oil of Oregano to Help Fight Your Sugar Cravings

Again, I think sugar cravings are less a sign of either low willpower or a cultivated taste than an indication of an imbalance in your body. Often, excess yeast within your system will cause you to crave sugar, even when you don't actually feel like eating it. So take an antiyeast formula to help overcome those cravings, and you may discover that you no longer have any interest in the Detox Detractors that may have been almost like an addiction for you.

Path C: The Fast Track Mix and Match

Path C is for all you Fat Flushers out there, who want to stay on your program while also taking advantage of the wonderful benefits of a one-day fast—not to mention the healing effects of adding enzymes, nucleotides, and probiotics to your diet.

Try to incorporate even more organic fruits and veggies into each of the three Fat Flush phases. You can also enhance your program with nucleotides by adding sardines into your menu plans three or four times a week or adding some yeast flakes or the blue-green algae (E3Live) to your morning or between-meal smoothies.

For probiotics, if you're on Phase 1 or 2, you can still be compliant with the program by incorporating sauerkraut instead of yogurt into your daily diet. Then in Phase 3 you might introduce yogurt. And if sauerkraut doesn't suit you, use the powdered probiotic (Flora-Key) from the Three-Day Sequel (page 125) first thing in the morning and in the evening in your Long Life Cocktail.

PATH C: THE FAST TRACK MIX AND MATCH

- *Eat all the Fast Track Mainstays.*

- *Avoid all Detox Detractors, except for your "legal" 1 cup of organic coffee or herbal coffee (such as Teeccino).*

- *Undertake the One-Day Detox Diet whenever you are transitioning from one phase to another. When you're ready to fast, regardless of which phase you are in, prepare your system by going back to at least one week of Phase 1, but skip the organic coffee, using the herbal coffee instead. Then follow up your One-Day Detox Diet by integrating the probiotic suggestions of the Seven-Day Prequel (as outlined in chapter 8 of this book) into your current phase.*

- *Buy at least 50 percent organic and make healthy choices according to the list given in this chapter.*

- *Continue to supplement your diet with the three formulas in the Fat Flush Kit.*

A Closer Look at Path C

Buy at Least 50 Percent Organic and Make Healthy Choices According to the Lists Given in This Chapter

If you've read *The Fat Flush Plan* closely, you already know how I feel about organic food! But I'll say it again: Detoxification is good for both your health *and* your weight loss. The more you're able to buy clean, healthy food, the better able you'll be to make the *Fat Flush Plan* work for you.

Continue to Supplement Your Diet with the Three Formulas in the Fat Flush Kit

The kit includes the Dieter's Multi, a balanced multivitamin for complete dietary insurance; a gamma linolenic acid (GLA) supplement to support weight loss; and a third special formula known as the Weight Loss Formula, which provides nutrients that support carbohydrate metabolism, fat burning, and liver health (see "Resources").

Recipes

Welcome to the recipe section. You will find that these surprisingly tasty and healthy detox recipes make it easy to integrate the Fast Track into everyday eating. To make things super convenient for you, many of the recipes have been identified as Prequel and/or Sequel friendly. I'm offering you recipes that feature liver-supporting ingredients (based on chapter 4) that have been shown to enhance cleansing and are protective for the liver. Specifically designed to be practical and deliciously nourishing to the liver, the liver-loving recipes emphasize foods such as cruciferous veggies, greens, cilantro, daikon, yeast flakes, and whey protein. In many of these recipes, you will find multiple liver-supporting substances like garlic, lemon juice, and cilantro.

Other recipes feature colon-caring choices. These are recipes that highlight colon support and cleansing elements such as high fiber flax, psyllium, oats and fruit. I include recipes for enhanced probiotic care that feature fermented foods such as sauerkraut and yogurt to support beneficial intestinal bacteria.

You will find that many of the recipes that appear in these sections contain multiple ingredients that will love your liver and care for your colon all in one, like Flaxy Chicken with Citrus Relish, which contains liver-supporting oranges, lime, and cilantro plus colon-caring high-fiber flaxseeds. Apple cider vinegar is woven into many recipes as well, like the Firecracker Slaw, which heads the recipe line-up.

Brand names are mentioned for specific products when they add significant taste, flavor, and health value. Do keep in mind that when salt is called for in these recipes, I would suggest you use plain old-fashioned Morton's canning and pickling salt, which does not contain any additives or mercury, which is a "hidden" ingredient in many so-called healthy sea salts in the marketplace.

Finally, for those who are taking the Fast Track to a higher level, you will find a method for growing your own organic sprouts and a whole repertoire of blended salads and even a special chlorophyll- and nucleotide-rich salsa.

THE LIVER-LOVING RECIPES
✳ Featuring the Crucial Crucifers ✳

FIRECRACKER SLAW
6 to 8 servings ✳ *prequel and sequel friendly*

If you are a single person, this makes enough slaw for about a week. This is a great way to integrate cabbage, refreshing lime, and enzyme-rich apple cider vinegar to purify your body from the inside out.

1 pound red and green cabbage, thinly sliced

2 medium carrots, thinly sliced

1 red bell pepper, finely chopped

1 green bell pepper, finely chopped

4 celery stalks, finely chopped

2 tablespoons fresh lime juice

2 tablespoons apple cider vinegar

4 teaspoons flaxseed oil

Cayenne, to taste

1/2 teaspoon celery seed

1. Combine all the ingredients in a large bowl with a lid.

2. Cover and shake.

3. Refrigerate for 4 to 6 hours to allow the flavors to develop, shaking periodically.

A CABBAGE SOUP
FOR ALL SEASONS
12 servings ✳ *prequel and sequel friendly*

This soup is great both warm for those chilly days and nights and cold for spring and summer. For a complete meal, add cooked chicken, turkey, or beef to the soup during the last 10 minutes of cooking.

1 head green cabbage
(tough leaves removed), coarsely sliced

1 cup sliced carrots

6 celery stalks, sliced

4 garlic cloves, minced

1 medium sweet onion, cut into chunks

1 medium zucchini,
halved and sliced

1 medium yellow squash,
halved and sliced

One 28-ounce can whole tomatoes
(Muir Glen)

One 28-ounce can diced tomatoes
(Muir Glen)

One 28-ounce can tomato puree
(Muir Glen)

½ cup minced fresh parsley

¼ cup minced fresh basil

¼ cup minced fresh chives

Salt or cayenne to taste

1. Place all the vegetables and the tomatoes, tomato puree, and 6 cups of filtered water in a large stockpot; bring to a boil, then cover.

2. Lower heat and simmer until the veggies are soft but not mushy, about 1 hour.

3. Add the herbs and salt or cayenne to taste.

STEAMED BROCCOLI AND CAULIFLOWER WITH PEA PODS

6 to 8 servings ✳ *prequel and sequel friendly*

E asy and light. This recipe makes enough for several days. It can be used for leftovers with scrambled eggs the next morning.

1 cup pea pods
2 medium shallots, diced
2 cups broccoli florets
1 cup cauliflower florets

1. Place 1 cup of filtered water in large pot and bring to a rolling boil.

2. Place a steamer in the pot and layer the pea pods, shallots, broccoli, and cauliflower.

3. Cover and steam until tender crisp, about 10 minutes.

BRUSSELS SPROUTS À L'ORANGE

4 to 6 servings ✳ *prequel and sequel friendly*

Aromatic spices like cinnamon, cloves, and ginger lend themselves surprisingly well to Brussels sprouts. If you have not been a Brussels sprouts fan, you may become converted.

1 pound Brussels sprouts, trimmed and halved

2 teaspoons grated orange rind

Dash of ground cinnamon

Dash of ground cloves

Dash of ground ginger

Salt to taste (optional)

1. Place 1 cup filtered water in a large pot and bring to a rolling boil.

2. Place a steamer in the pot and add the Brussels sprouts. Cover and steam until tender crisp, 10 to 12 minutes.

3. Add the orange rind, cover, and steam for another 3 minutes.

4. Sprinkle on the cinnamon, cloves, ginger, and salt, if using. Remove from the heat.

LIVER-LOVING RECIPES
※ *Featuring Glorious Greens* ※

GARLICKY GREENS WITH GINGER AND LEMON
4 servings ※ *prequel and sequel friendly*

G reens are cleansing and full of liver-loving chlorophyll, especially those bitter greens. To take out the bitterness, always use a bit of salt when cooking. The salt sweetens up the greens quite nicely, removing the bitter taste.

3 tablespoons low-sodium chicken broth
(Pacific Organic) or olive oil

1 large bunch (about 1 pound) greens
(kale, chard, mustard, beet greens, or collards),
cut crosswise with stems removed

2 garlic cloves, minced

1/8 teaspoon powdered ginger

Pinch of salt

2 tablespoons fresh lemon juice

1. Heat the broth or oil in a sauté pan over medium heat.

2. Add the greens, garlic, ginger, and salt, stirring until the greens wilt, about 1 1/2 minutes.

3. Remove from the heat and drizzle on the lemon juice.

LAYERED RAINBOW SALAD WITH BROCCOLI SPROUTS

4 servings ✳ *prequel and sequel friendly*

Here's an all-in-one salad your liver will surely love for a light lunch or dinner. This will last for several meals in the fridge and gets better every day. It is packed with purifying greens, antioxidant-rich broccoli sprouts, betaine-rich crimson beets, and even cilantro.

1 cup mixed salad greens

1 cup baby greens, stems removed

1/2 cup watercress

2 tablespoons flaxseed or olive oil

1/4 teaspoon dried mustard

1 teaspoon minced fresh garlic

1 tablespoon apple cider vinegar

1/2 cup minced fresh cilantro

2 tablespoons fresh lemon juice

1/2 cup broccoli sprouts (Brocco Sprouts)

1/2 cup shredded beets

1/2 cup shredded carrots

1 hard-boiled egg, sliced, for garnish

Fresh dill weed, for garnish

1. Combine the mixed greens, baby greens, and watercress in a large salad bowl; set aside.

2. In a small bowl, whisk the oil, mustard, garlic, vinegar, cilantro, and lemon juice.

3. Pour the dressing mixture over the greens and toss lightly.

4. Add the broccoli sprouts. Layer on the beets and then the carrots.

5. Garnish with the eggs and dill weed.

6. Cover the bowl and keep in the fridge until ready to serve.

PESTO PRESTO CILANTRO

makes 1 cup ✳ *prequel and sequel friendly*

Just a couple of teaspoons a day will keep those heavy metals away! Great with salads or as a dip for a variety of freshly cut veggies. Freezes well in self-sealing plastic bags.

1½ cups packed fresh cilantro
6 tablespoons flaxseed oil or olive oil
2 tablespoons fresh lemon juice
2 garlic cloves, minced

1. Place the cilantro and oil in a food processor. Process until the cilantro is well chopped.

2. Add the lemon juice and garlic. Process again until a paste is formed, scraping down the sides of the processor's bowl as needed. Serve right away or cover and refrigerate.

CUCUMBER CILANTRO SALSA

4 servings ✳ *prequel and sequel friendly*

Don't like to fuss? No problem. Here's an oh-so-easy and refreshing topping for scrambled eggs and a dip for fresh veggies. I like this plain by the spoonful out of the fridge. This is the perfect Liver-Loving addition to any wrap.

1 large cucumber, peeled and shredded

1 large tomato, chopped

2 tablespoons minced red onion

½ teaspoon ground cumin

2 tablespoons chopped fresh cilantro

1 garlic clove, minced (optional)

1. Combine all the ingredients in a small bowl. Toss lightly.

2. Cover and chill for at least 1 hour before serving.

LIVER-LOVING RECIPES
✳ Featuring Cleansing Citrus ✳

GINGERY LIMEADE
Makes 4 cups ✳ *prequel and sequel friendly*

This, of course, is a variation on good old-fashioned lemonade. I have used this for company on many occasions, and it is a winner. The addition of Stevia Plus for sweetening cuts down on carbs and calories. You can always use lemons instead of the limes.

Juice, pulp, and grated rind of 3 to 4 limes
2 tablespoons finely grated fresh ginger
1/4 teaspoon Stevia Plus, or to taste

1. Combine 4 cups filtered water with all the ingredients in a tall pitcher. Mix or whisk well.
2. Cover and chill before serving.

LIVER-LOVING RECIPES
✳ *Featuring Daikon* ✳

DELIGHTFUL DAIKON RELISH
4 servings ✳ *prequel and sequel friendly*

Here's a tasty way to dress up fish, lamb, or beef.

½ cup shredded daikon radish
¼ teaspoon ground ginger
½ teaspoon minced fresh parsley

1. Place the daikon in a small bowl.

2. Sprinkle with the ginger and parsley.

LIVER-LOVING RECIPES
❋ *Featuring Artichokes, Whey Protein, and Yeast Flakes* ❋

ABSOLUTELY ARTICHOKE SOUP
2 servings ❋ *prequel and sequel friendly*

This is absolutely delicious, and your liver (not to mention your family) will agree!

1 tablespoon chicken broth
(Pacific Organic) or olive oil

1 small onion, minced

4 garlic cloves, minced

One 14-ounce can artichokes,
rinsed, drained, and chopped

2 cups broth or stock

½ teaspoon dried parsley

½ teaspoon dried basil

½ teaspoon dried oregano

Salt to taste (optional)

Cayenne to taste (optional)

Fresh lemon juice to taste (optional)

1. Heat the broth or oil in a stockpot over medium heat.

2. Sauté the onion and garlic until translucent.

3. Stir in the artichokes, broth, and herbs. Add the salt, cayenne, and/or lemon juice, if using.

4. Cover and simmer for 30 minutes.

WHEY DELISH PANCAKES

makes 6 to 8 (3-inch) pancakes ✳ *prequel and sequel friendly*

What a whey to begin your day! These pancakes are terrific with some added fruit or a tablespoon or two of milled or ground flaxseeds for added tender loving colon care. The flaxseeds taste somewhere between toasted wheat germ and ground-up walnuts.

4 eggs
1 scoop whey (Fat Flush Whey vanilla)
1 teaspoon ground cinnamon
1/4 teaspoon ground cloves
Olive oil spray

1. Place all the ingredients in a blender and blend until well mixed. (Note that the batter will be a bit thin and runny.)

2. Heat a nonstick pan, and spray with the olive oil spray to lightly coat the pan.

3. Spoon the batter (about 3 tablespoons) into the pan, spreading it to create a pancake by gently shaking the pan.

4. Flip the pancake when the edges are lightly browned. Continue to cook for a few seconds longer.

5. Remove the pancake from the pan and place on a flat surface.

6. Repeat until all the batter has been used up.

JICAMA STIX

4 servings ✳ *prequel and sequel friendly*

Jicama is the best-kept dieter's secret because it is high in potassium and has a crisp, sweet flavor that's a bit like water chestnuts. Here it gives us a crunchy excuse to snack and enjoy nutritional yeast flakes, which are rich in easily absorbable B vitamins. Great for lunch-box treats and between-meal snacks.

1 medium jicama, peeled and cut into thin strips
1 tablespoon nutritional yeast flakes (Kal or Lewis Labs)
1/2 teaspoon ground cumin
1/2 teaspoon dried dill
1/4 teaspoon salt
2 tablespoons flaxseed or rice bran oil

1. Place the jicama in a small bowl and set aside.

2. In another bowl, mix the remaining ingredients together.

3. Pour the yeast mixture over the jicama and stir to coat.

COLON-CARING RECIPES
* *Featuring High-Fiber Psyllium, Flax,* *
Oatmeal, Pears, and Berries

SPICED SEEDS
1 serving * *prequel and sequel friendly*

This mixture of high-fiber psyllium and flax can be used as a seasoning or sprinkled over salads or steamed veggies.

1 teaspoon powdered psyllium husks
1 tablespoon milled flaxseed (FiProFlax)
1 tablespoon ground fennel seeds
1 tablespoon ground anise seeds

Mix all ingredients together in a small bowl.

FLAXY CHICKEN WITH CITRUS RELISH

4 servings ✳ *prequel and sequel friendly*

little bit more involved in terms of time. But for those who love to cook, this recipe is loaded with fiber and is good for your waistline, too.

Citrus Relish

2 tablespoons grated orange rind

1 cup fresh orange juice

1 teaspoon grated lime rind

2 tablespoons fresh lime juice

1 tablespoon arrowroot

1 orange, cut and sectioned like a grapefruit

1 cup diced seeded cucumber

1/4 cup chopped scallions

1/4 cup finely diced yellow bell pepper

1/4 cup finely diced red bell pepper

2 tablespoons chopped cilantro

Salt to taste

Cayenne to taste

Chicken

Olive oil spray

1 egg, beaten

1/4 cup Dijon mustard

Salt (optional)

Cayenne to taste

1/2 cup milled or ground flaxseeds (FiProFlax)

4 boneless chicken breast halves, skin removed

1 1/2 tablespoons olive oil

Citrus Relish

1. Combine the orange rind, orange juice, lime rind, lime juice, and arrowroot in a small saucepan.

2. Simmer over medium heat until bubbly and thick.

3. Cool.

4. In small bowl, mix the remaining relish ingredients. Stir in the orange and lime mixture until well blended.

5. Let the mixture stand, covered, for at least 1 hour so flavors can marry.

Chicken

1. Preheat the oven to 350°. Lightly coat a baking sheet with olive oil spray.

2. Place the beaten egg in a shallow dish.

3. Combine the mustard, salt (if using), cayenne, and flaxseeds in a pie plate.

4. Dip the chicken breasts into the beaten egg, and then dredge in the flaxseeds, coating all sides well.

5. Place the chicken on the baking sheet; drizzle with the olive oil.

6. Bake 35 minutes, until chicken is cooked through and juices run clear.

7. Serve the chicken topped with the Citrus Relish.

SWEETIE PIE FLAX
SNACK CRACKERS

36 2-inch square crackers ✳ *prequel and sequel friendly*

This recipe is versatile and satisfying. You can get creative by substituting 1 tablespoon of minced garlic for the cinnamon, cloves, whey, and stevia. Or how about 1/4 cup chopped olives and red peppers, 2 teaspoons of chives, or 1 tablespoon of cayenne or chili powder instead?

Olive oil spray
1/2 cup milled or ground flaxseeds (FiProFlax)
2 teaspoons ground cinnamon
1/2 teaspoon ground cloves
1 teaspoon whey (Fat Flush Whey vanilla)
Dash powdered stevia
1 teaspoon ground allspice

1. Preheat the oven to 250°F. Spray a cookie sheet with olive oil spray.

2. Mix the flaxseeds, cinnamon, cloves, whey, stevia, and allspice together.

3. Add enough filtered water (about 1/4 cup) to form the mixture into a ball.

4. Place the dough between two pieces of wax paper. Roll very thin.

5. Remove the paper and score the dough into 2-inch-square crackers.

6. Bake 30 to 40 minutes, until the crackers pull up from the cookie sheet.

7. Store in cool place or pantry.

Tip: These can be baked on a baking stone.

FIBER HIGH TRUFFLES

Makes 30 to 36 truffles ✳ *prequel and sequel friendly*

S pecifically designed for those who want their fiber but do not have to lose weight. Kids love this recipe too.

1/2 cup natural peanut butter

1/3 cup unheated natural honey

3/4 cup whey (Fat Flush Whey Protein vanilla)

1/2 teaspoon ground cinnamon

1/2 cup coarsely ground macadamia nuts

2 tablespoons milled or ground flaxseeds

3 tablespoons toasted sesame seeds

1 cup Uncle Sam's Cereal

1/4 cup raisins

1/4 cup chopped unsweetened dried apricots

1/4 cup crushed toasted sliced almonds

Carob powder for dusting

1. Place the peanut butter, honey, whey, cinnamon, macadamia nuts, flaxseeds, sesame seeds, cereal, raisins, and apricots in a food processor fitted with a steel knife. Process using on-and-off turns until well combined and the mixture holds together.

2. Let the mixture rest for 10 minutes.

3. Line a baking sheet with wax paper.

4. Form the mixture into 1-inch balls. Roll each ball in the crushed almonds, pressing to adhere.

5. Place the carob powder in a small sieve. Sprinkle the truffles lightly with the carob, rolling the balls to evenly cover the surface.

6. Let the truffles rest on the baking sheet for 10 minutes.

7. Refrigerate in an airtight container.

Tip: Freezes well.

PEARFECT MUESLI
1 serving ✳ *prequel and sequel friendly*

This dish is my Fast Track version of the famous Bircher-Benner Muesli from Switzerland. This is suitable for people who want their fiber but do not need to lose weight.

4 tablespoons filtered water

2 tablespoons old-fashioned
rolled oats (not instant)

Juice of ½ lemon

1 tablespoon whey in 1 tablespoon of
filtered water (Fat Flush Whey vanilla)

1 medium pear

1 tablespoon unprocessed, raw honey

2 tablespoons milled or ground flaxseeds (FiProFlax) or

chopped nuts of your choice

1. Soak the oatmeal overnight in 4 tablespoons of filtered water.

2. In the morning, add the lemon juice and the whey mixture, blending well.

3. Shred the pear into the mixture.

4. Add the honey and flaxseeds or nuts and stir. Eat at once.

MORNING-AFTER
PUFFY APPLE FLAXCAKE

1 serving ✳ *prequel and sequel friendly*

T his is definitely the breakfast of choice for the morning after
the One-Day Detox Diet. You can use this, of course, anytime in the program.

1 to 2 tablespoons filtered water

1 egg

2 tablespoons shredded apple

3 tablespoons milled or ground flaxseeds

1 teaspoon Stevia Plus

1/8 to 1/2 teaspoon of cinnamon

Olive oil spray

1. Whisk the egg, apple, flaxseeds, and stevia together with 1 to
    2 tablespoons of filtered water in a small bowl.

2. Lightly coat an omelet pan with olive oil spray and heat over
    medium heat.

3. Pour the egg mixture into the pan and cook until the bottom of
    the flaxcake is solid enough to flip, 3 to 4 minutes.

4. Carefully flip the flaxcake, cooking until done, about 1 minute.

5. Sprinkle with the cinnamon and serve.

PROBIOTIC-POWERING RECIPES
✳ *Featuring Sauerkraut and Yogurt* ✳

ANN LOUISE'S HOMEMADE SAUERKRAUT
Makes 1 quart ✳ *sequel friendly*

The key to this sauerkraut recipe is that it maintains its naturally occurring enzymes and microflora. This is an uncooked rendition that is quite tasty.

2 cups shredded red cabbage

2 cups shredded green cabbage

1 teaspoon dried mustard

1 teaspoon caraway seeds

1 teaspoon salt

1 garlic clove, minced

2 tablespoons fresh lemon juice

1 cup filtered water

1. In a glass container with a cover, combine the cabbages, mustard, caraway seeds, and salt.

2. In a separate small bowl combine the garlic, lemon juice, and 1 cup filtered water. Then pour the mixture over the cabbage.

3. Cover tightly. Set aside and keep the cabbage at room temperature for at least 3 days, shaking occasionally.

SAUERKRAUT
STUFFED TOMATOES

4 servings ✳ *sequel friendly*

Sauerkraut and tomatoes make a surprisingly tasty combination.

1 cup sauerkraut (Ann Louise's Homemade Sauerkraut,
page 204, Rejuvenative Foods, Eden, or Cascadian Farm)

½ teaspoon ground coriander

½ teaspoon poppy seeds

¼ teaspoon dried mustard

1 teaspoon minced chives

4 large firm tomatoes

1. Mix the sauerkraut, coriander, poppy seeds, mustard, and chives together in a small bowl.

2. Cut off the tops of the tomatoes about one quarter of the way down; save the tops. Scoop out the pulp and drain the tomatoes.

3. Stuff the tomatoes with the sauerkraut mixture.

4. Replace the tops when serving.

FRUITY YOGURT

1 serving ✳ *sequel friendly*

This is a lovely "cultured" snack or dessert, providing beneficial bacteria as well as colon-caring flaxseeds. It makes a good topping or filling for Whey Delish Pancakes (page 195).

1 cup plain organic yogurt
1 cup mixed berries
1 tablespoon milled or ground flaxseeds
Dash of ground ginger
Dash of ground cinnamon

1. Combine the yogurt, berries, and flaxseeds in a small bowl.

2. Spoon into parfait glass.

3. Sprinkle with the ginger and cinnamon. Chill before serving.

SPROUT-IT-YOURSELF METHOD

You can certainly buy high-quality organic sprouts in a health-food store or even in a good grocery store, but if you'd like to make your own, here's how to start:

- Pour seeds into a clean glass jar whose mouth is wide enough to enable you to get the grown sprouts out. For small seeds, you should just cover the bottom of the jar; for large seeds, fill the jar about one eighth full.

- Cover the seeds with room temperature filtered water. You want to add about two or three times the volume of the seeds.

- Soak small seeds for four to six hours and large ones for eight to twelve hours. Change the water for large seeds at least twice, and don't let them soak more than twelve hours, or they might ferment.

- Cover the jar with a sprouting lid, which will let the water drain out while the sprouts stay in (you can buy one in your health food store). Put the jar upside down in a position that allows oxygen to enter the jar, in a place where the temperature will stay around 70°F. Rinse your sprouts two or three times a day. Avoid excess moisture or insufficient air, or you'll end up with moldy sprouts. But don't let them get too dry or they'll die.

- After a few days, make sure they're in indirect sunlight for about six hours. Then harvest your bounty. The sprouts' "tails" should be about one and a half times as long as the seeds.

- Store any uneaten sprouts in your fridge, and rinse them every three days. They should keep about a week.

  Consider sprouting broccoli, clover, radish, sunflower, fenu-greek, alfalfa, buckwheat, clover, mustard, or sunflower sprouts, which are both nutritious and easy to grow.

BLENDED SALAD RECIPES

It is very important that the veggies in these blended salads are from organic vegetables. The last thing you want in your system is liquefied pesticides, sprays, and fungicides.

GODDESS GREENS
1 serving

2 cups mixed green lettuce
2 celery stalks
½ cup spinach
1 cucumber
½ garlic clove, minced (optional)
Juice of ½ lemon or lime

1. Cut the lettuce, celery, spinach, and cucumber in small pieces.

2. Place the veggies and garlic, if using, in a food processor or blender. Process or blend until liquefied.

3. Add the lemon or lime juice.

4. Drink immediately.

DANDY GREENS
1 serving

2 cups romaine lettuce
1/2 cup dandelion greens
1 cup radish sprouts
1/2 garlic clove, minced (optional)
Juice of 1/2 lemon or lime

1. Cut the lettuce and greens in small pieces.

2. Place the greens, sprouts, and garlic, if using, in a food processor or blender. Process or blend until liquefied.

3. Add the lemon or lime juice.

4. Drink immediately.

SPINACH SURPRISE
1 serving

2 cups spinach
½ scallion
1 cup alfalfa sprouts
½ garlic clove, minced
Juice of ½ lemon or lime

1. Cut the spinach and scallion in small pieces.

2. Place the veggies, sprouts, and garlic, if using, in a food processor or blender. Process or blend until liquefied.

3. Add the lemon or lime juice.

4. Drink immediately.

PARSLEY FRESH
1 serving

1 cup mixed leafy greens

1 scallion

2 slices red bell pepper

$\frac{1}{2}$ tomato

$\frac{1}{2}$ cucumber

4 parsley sprigs

$\frac{1}{2}$ garlic clove, minced

Juice of $\frac{1}{2}$ lemon or lime

1. Cut the greens, scallion, bell pepper, tomato, and cucumber in small pieces.

2. Place the veggies, parsley, and garlic in a food processor or blender. Process or blend until liquefied.

3. Add the lemon or lime juice.

4. Drink immediately.

STRING BEAN DREAM
1 serving

2 cups romaine lettuce
1 cup string beans
1 small zucchini
1/2 cucumber
1/2 garlic clove, minced
Juice of 1/2 lemon or lime

1. Cut the lettuce, beans, zucchini, and cucumber in small pieces.

2. Place the veggies and garlic in a food processor or blender. Process or blend until liquefied.

3. Add the lemon or lime juice.

4. Drink immediately.

SPROUT SUPREME
1 serving

2 cups romaine lettuce
2 scallions
1 tomato
1 cup alfalfa sprouts
½ garlic clove, minced
Juice of ½ lemon or lime

1. Cut the lettuce, scallions, and tomato in small pieces.

2. Place the veggies, sprouts, and garlic in a food processor or blender. Process or blend until liquefied.

3. Add the lemon or lime juice.

4. Drink immediately.

E3LIVE SALSA
Makes 4¹/₂ cups

No, this isn't a new dance step, but this E3Live superfood will surely give you a kick. It's a living source of chlorophyll, nucleotides, vitamins, minerals, enzymes, and phytonutrients.

5 large tomatoes, coarsely chopped

3 tablespoons finely chopped cilantro

1 to 2 jalapeño peppers, seeded and minced

2 garlic cloves, minced

1 small onion, finely chopped

2 tablespoons fresh lime juice

Salt to taste (optional)

1 small avocado, finely chopped

1 tablespoon E3Live

Combine all ingredients in a large bowl and mix well.

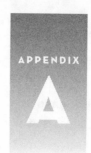

APPENDIX

A

Resources

SPECIALTY DETOX FOODS AND DIETARY SUPPLEMENTS

**The Official Fast Track Web site is
www.fasttrackdetox.com**

Want to become a Fast Tracker but are looking for support? We feature an online support group for every step of the program. Plus, here's the ultimate resource for many of your Fast Track specialty detox foods and dietary supplements that are mentioned in the Seven-Day Prequel, One-Day Detox Diet, Three-Day Sequel, and Taking It to the Next Level chapters. This site is also a source for the Doulton Ceramic Water Filter and the Fat Flush Whey, one of the only commercially available unheated, undenatured whey protein concentrate powders on the market, which is made from milk that is hormone-treatment free. Other Fast Track supplements available include the Fast Detox Diet Kit (Super-GI Cleanse, the Liver-Lovin' Formula, and Flora-Key), hydrochloric acid with pepsin and ox bile, FiProFlax, Men's FiProFlax, LiverCare, AF Betafood, Dr. Ohhira's Probiotics 12 Plus, copper-free female multiple, iron-free male multiple, Time C, vitamin E, Oxy-Key, omega-3 fish oil, GLA-90, Weight Loss Formula, The Adrenal Formula, Y-C Cleanse, and the Fat Flush Kit for ongoing weight loss support and liver health. The Fat Flush Kit consists of a Dieter's Multi, the GLA-90s, the Weight Loss Formula.

Do-It-Yourself Tests

To complement your detox journey, the following do-it-yourself tests access heavy metal toxicity, parasite and yeast infestation, and hormone imbalances.

Hair analysis. This analysis includes a full report, up to twenty pages, which graphically shows the levels of thirty-two major minerals and six toxic metals in the body. Each mineral is fully evaluated in terms of its relationship with other minerals. There is also a complete discussion in regard to disease tendencies based on mineral levels and ratios.

Parasite test kit. The purged stool sample is collected in the privacy of your home and is sent directly to the Parasitology Testing Center in Arizona, one of the premier parasitology laboratories in the country. Your sample is examined for over a dozen protozoa, fifteen types of worms, plus the common yeasts (including *Candida albicans* and fungi spores).

Saliva hormone test. Unlike blood tests, which do not measure bio-available hormone activity, saliva testing is considered to be the most accurate measure of free, bio-available hormonal activity. This personal hormone evaluation can be used to profile up to six hormones, including estradiol, estriol, progesterone, testosterone, DHEA, and cortisol. Your personal results and a personal letter of recommendation from my office are mailed directly to your home.

Sprouts and Algae

BroccoSprouts
877–747–1277
www.broccosprouts.com

Broccoli sprouts are the only product that guarantees a consistent level of sulforaphane GS, a natural compound found in broccoli and other cruciferous plants that supports the body's own antioxidant function. Developed by scientists at Johns Hopkins University School of Medicine, broccoli sprouts and sprout blends are now available in supermarkets around the country.

E3Live
Vision Inc.
P.O. Box N
Klamath Falls, OR 97601
EST: 888–800–7070; PST: 888–233–1441; international: 541–273–2212; fax: 541–273–9213
www.E3Live.com

E3Live markets a line of high-quality, wild blue-green algae with unique health properties from Upper Klamath Lake in Oregon. The algae is available frozen or in a dried powder form. This company also markets truffles filled with algae, which make unique and healthy gifts.

ONE-DAY DETOX DIET SUPPLIES

Organic Unsweetened Cranberry Juice

Lakewood 100% Organic Pure Cranberry Juice
www.lakewoodjuices.com
info@floridabottling.com

Lakewood seeks to deliver to the marketplace top-quality fruit products that are manufactured under guidelines of integrity and respect for our environment. One-hundred-percent organic!

Water

HydroPro/Aqua Rush Water
Xtreme Technologies, Inc.
1620B Northwest Blvd., Suite 300
Coeur d'Alene, ID 83814
888–424–7874
www.hydropro.us

When it comes to bottled water, I like HydroPro/Aqua Rush Water. It's processed with patented technology that helps create optimum hydration.

Organic and Nonirradiated Herbs and Spices

Triple Leaf, Inc.
P.O. Box 421572
San Francisco, CA 94142
800–552–7448; 650–588–8406
www.tripleleaf-tea.com

A source of organic and nonirradiated cinnamon, nutmeg, and ginger.

Frontier Natural Products Co-op
P.O. Box 299
3021 Seventy-Eighth St.
Norway, IA 52318
800–669–3275; fax: 800–717–4372
www.frontiercoop.com

A source of organic and nonirradiated cinnamon, nutmeg, and ginger. All Simply Organic products are produced under strict organic guidelines, without irradiation, genetically modified organisms, or harmful pesticides, herbicides, or synthetic fertilizers. Products are certified organic by Quality Assurance International.

Conscious Light Botanicals
7081 East Fifth Ave.
Scottsdale, AZ 85251
480–970–6157; 866–970–6157; fax: 480–970–6156
www.consciouslight.com

A source of organic and nonirradiated cinnamon, nutmeg, and ginger.

Gold Mine Natural Foods
7805 Arjon's Dr.
San Diego, CA 92126
800–475–3663
www.goldminenaturalfood.com
A source of organic and nonirradiated cinnamon, nutmeg, and ginger as well as many other high-quality products.

Natural Lifestyle Supplies Mail Order Market
16 Lookout Dr.
Asheville, NC 28804–3330
800–752–2775
www.natural-lifestyle.com

A source of organic and nonirradiated cinnamon, nutmeg, and ginger as well as many other fine products.

Spice Hunter
184 Suburban Rd.
San Luis Obispo, CA 93401
800–444–3061
www.spicehunter.com

A source of organic and nonirradiated herbs and spices and many exotic blends.

Natural Grocers

Wild Oats Natural Marketplace
800–494–WILD; 303–440–5220
www.wildoats.com

The Wild Oats family of natural food stores, including Wild Oats, Alfalfa's, and Nature's Northwest, are convenient sources in many of the larger cities for organic produce, organically raised beef without antibiotics or steroids, free-range chicken and turkey, bison, organic and hormone-free dairy, and omega-3 enriched eggs. Many also carry the highest quality ingredients for the One-Day Detox Diet Miracle Juice, such as Lakewood Organic cranberry juice, Knudsen's cranberry juice, and Tree of Life cranberry concentrate as well as non-irradiated and organic herbs and spices from brands like Frontier Natural Products Co-op and Spice Hunters.

Whole Foods Market
512–477–4455
www.wholefoods.com

Whole Foods is now the largest chain of natural food stores nationwide. They offer organic produce, organically raised beef without antibiotics or steroids, free-range chicken and turkey, bison, organic and hormone-free dairy, and omega-3 enriched eggs. They also carry unsweetened cranberry juice and nonirradiated and organic herbs and spices.

Trader Joe's
800–746–7857
www.traderjoes.com

Trader Joe's is one of the best-kept secrets in specialty retail grocery stores. They offer better prices than health food supermarkets because they buy direct from suppliers. You can often find organic produce, organic beef, free-range poultry, and omega-3 enriched eggs and lots of other surprises. They often carry unsweetened cranberry juice under their own Trader Joe's label.

Organic Brands

Rejuvenative Foods
800–805–7957

www.rejuvenative.com

Rejuvenative Foods Raw Sauerkraut is a handcrafted 100 percent fresh cultured vegetable, high in fiber and low in fat, which is hand-made with great care to provide a flavorful, rich source of enzymes and lactobacilli.

Earthbound Farm
800–690–3200

www.ebfarm.com

This is the largest supplier of fresh organic fruits and veggies. Their Grab-&-Go organic salad kits are convenient.

Earth's Best
800–434–4246

www.earthsbest.com

An organic baby-food company that makes cereals, pureed foods, juices, and bars with only organic ingredients.

Eden Foods
888–441–3336

www.edenfoods.com

Eden Foods was the first certified organic food-processing facility in North America.

Health Valley
800–434–4246
www.healthvalley.com

From soups to crackers and even pet foods, Health Valley is noted for their all-natural ingredients without artificial colors, flavors, or preservatives.

Horizon Organic
888–494–3020
www.horizonorganic.com

Horizon Organic boasts a full line of certified organic milk and other dairy, egg, and juice products. The company strongly believes in the importance of organic agriculture, with an emphasis on high-quality dairy and juice products.

Nancy's Cultured Dairy & Soy
541–689–2911
www.nancysyogurt.com

Organic Valley
888–444–6455
www.organicvalley.com

This company includes more than 600 farms in seventeen states that produce organic milk, cheese, eggs, butter, meat, and juice.

Stonyfield Farm
800–776–2697
www.stonyfield.com

This is the largest producer of organic yogurt in the world.

Organic Frozen Foods

Cascadian Frozen Foods
800–624–4123
www.cfarm.com

Cascadian Farm has become a leading grower, manufacturer, and distributor of a wide range of delicious organic products, from frozen fruit (including blueberries, strawberries, raspberries, sliced peaches, cherries, harvest berries, and blackberries) to breakfast cereal. The company's products are sold throughout the United States in natural food stores and select supermarkets. They are also a source of organic spinach.

Stahlbush Island Farms, Inc.
541–757–1497
www.stahlbush.com

Premium processors of fruit and vegetable purees and individually quick-frozen vegetables and fruits. They also offer custom processing of organic, sustainable, and conventional fruits and vegetables in a kosher-certified facility.

Healthy Fish

Sardines
Sardines from Crown Prince and Bela are often carried in finer health food stores. But, if not, here is the contact information for these two fine brands:

Crown Prince
707–766–8575
www.crownprince.com

Crown Prince offers wild-caught boneless and skinless sardines. You can also find mackerel and kippers.

Bela-Olhao
508–401–0001; 866–4–MY–BELLA; fax: 508–401–0008; info@bluegalleon.com; www.mytunafish.com

Bela-Olhao also carries sardines as well as small tuna steaks, which are very low in mercury, unlike the bigger tuna.

Wild Salmon
The following Web sites carry wild salmon, a rich source of the omega-3 fatty acids. Some, such as www.tunatuna.com and www.sea maiden.com, have tested their fish and have found that they are virtually mercury free.

Copper River Seafoods
888–622–1197
www.copperriverseafood.com

Kasilof Fish Company
800–322–7552
www.ilovesalmon.com

Alaska Wild Salmon Company
866–463–3458
www.alaskawildsalmoncompany.com

EcoFish
603–430–0101
www.ecofish.com

Fishing Vessel St. Jude
425–378–0680
www.tunatuna.com

Cinda's Sea Maiden's Harvest
503–245–1596
www.seamaiden.com

East Point Seafood Market
888–317–8459
www.eastpointseafood.com

HEALTHY BEEF

Grass-raised beef is becoming more popular and sometimes can be found in local food co-ops and health food stores.

Eat Wild
866–453–8489
www.eatwild.com

The clearinghouse for information about pasture-based farming. This Web site provides a state-by-state directory to help you locate grass-fed beef, lamb, bison, poultry, and dairy products from pastured animals. For more information, call.

Great Beef
www.greatbeef.com
cimarron@greatbeef.com

The natural beef growers network. This Web site provides an excellent source of free-range or pasture-fed livestock and poultry and will hook you up with local producers in Arizona, California, Colorado, Iowa, Minnesota, Missouri, Nebraska, Nevada, Oregon, Pennsylvania, Tennessee, Texas, and Virginia.

Eat Well Guide
www.iatp.org/eatwell

This Web site includes state-by-state listings of meat that is raised without antibiotics.

Grassland Beef
877–383–0051
www.grasslandbeef.com

This Web site provides a listing of beef with a high omega-3 content that is certified by the University of Iowa.

FAST TRACK TOOLS OF THE TRADE

Vita-Mix Corporation
Household Division
8615 Usher Rd.
Cleveland, OH 44138
800–848–2649
www.vitamix.com

Unlike other juicers, this high-speed, multipurpose machine makes low-glycemic total juices, which contain the fiber, vitamins, and minerals that extraction juicers remove. It also replaces a blender, food processor, ice crusher, grain grinder, and several other appliances. No ordinary blender can even begin to compete with the powerful Vita-Mix.

Tribest Corporation
14109 Pontlavoy Ave.
Santa Fe Springs, CA 90670
Voice: 562–623–7150; fax: 562–623–7160; 888–254–7336
www.tribest.com

Tribest carries a convenient easy-to-use automatic sprouter called the Tribest Freshlife Sprouter, which can produce sprouts in as little as four days. They also offer the compact and convenient Tribest Personal Blender, which is ideal for smoothies when you are on the road.

Sproutman's Automatic Sprouter
P.O. Box 1100
Great Barrington, MA 01230
413–528–5200; fax: 413–528–5201
www.sproutman.com

This automatic salad grower is an easy and economical way to provide your whole family with fresh, living sprouts—the world's most nutritious vegetables. The company also specializes in organically grown, pesticide-free, sprouting-grade seeds.

NUTRITIONALLY ORIENTED ORGANIZATIONS

American College for Advancement in Medicine (ACAM)
23121 Verdugo Dr.
Suite 204
Laguna Hills, CA 92653
800–532–3688; 949–583–7666
www.acam.org

The professional members of this organization are highly skilled in nutrition and various protocols mentioned in this book. This is a good start for contacting a doctor-member who can perform the Heidelberg test, which assesses gastric acidity and the need for HCl.

American Academy of Environmental Medicine
7701 E. Kellogg, Suite 625
Wichita, KS 67207
316–684–5500; fax: 316–684–5709; 316–684–5500
www.aaem.com

Like ACAM, the American Academy of Environmental Medicine is a professional organization that includes doctor-members who are nutritionally oriented.

NUTRITIONALLY ORIENTED DENTISTS

Hal A. Huggins, D.D.S., M.S.
Matrix, Inc.
5082 List Dr.
Colorado Springs, CO 80919
866–948–4638; 719–593–9616; fax: 719–548–8220
email@hugnet.com; www.DrHuggins.com

Dr. Huggins is a pioneer in correcting imbalances in body chemistry created by dental materials. He believes that many incurable diseases such as multiple sclerosis, amyotrophic lateral sclerosis, Parkinson's disease, Alzheimer's disease, lupus, leukemia, and sudden heart attack can be linked to incompatible dental materials, bridges, crowns, root canals, cavitations, and impacted wisdom teeth. His Web site provides you with key information about the hazards of mercury, nickel, root canals, and cavitations as well as offers books and video tapes (such as *The Coors Study—A Landmark in Dental Research*).

SPAS AND RETREATS

THEGREENHOUSE Destination Spa
Box 1141
Arlington, TX 76004
817–640–4000
www.thegreenhousespa.net

THEGREENHOUSE Day Spa
127 E. 57th St.
New York City, NY 10022
212–644–4449

THEGREENHOUSE is the exclusive home of The Fat Flush Residential and Spa Spectacular programs outside of Arlington, Texas. THEGREENHOUSE has been the spa of choice for women from all over the world, including first ladies, international royalty, supermodels, and movie and television personalities, since its inception in 1965. The Destination Spa offers the Fast Track program.

LABORATORIES FOR TESTING

Your Future Health
P.O. Box 1369
Tavares, FL 32778
877–468–6934
www.yourfuturehealth.com

Since 1976, this laboratory for accessing nutrient levels has specialized in blood testing and customized nutritional analysis. They also provide a unique essential fatty acid test that evaluates key essential fatty acids for health and longevity.

Scientific Health Solutions, Inc.
1621 N. Circle Dr.
Colorado Springs, CO 80909
800–331–2303

This laboratory specializes in serum biocompatibility testing in which the least-toxic replacement dental materials can be assessed. The report—which is over thirty pages in length and has "Highly Reactive," "Moderately Reactive," and "Least Reactive" categories—lists over 1,000 different dental products, including composite fillings, crown materials, bridge materials, cements, denture materials, and other materials. Nearly all reports have some materials in the least-reactive category from which the dentist may choose.

Jakaré
P.O. Box 10124
Bozeman, MT 59719–0124
877–525–2731
www.jakare.com

Jakaré provides skin care products made weekly. They specialize in lavender-scented lotions, potpourris, bath salts, and soaps.

Dr. Hauschka Skin Care
888–295–6802
www.essentialdayspa.com/Dr-Hauschka-Face-Care.htm

Available in many fine health food stores, Dr. Hauschka's products are pure and good for very dry skin.

Avalon Natural Products
800–227–5120
www.avalonorganics.com

Doctors Choice, Naturally
866–698–1581
www.doctorschoicenaturally.com

This company carries excellent organic hair and skin care products.

Fast Track Detox Methods

High Tech Health
800–794–5355
www.hightechhealth.com

This company offers Thermal Life Far Infrared Saunas, which promote detoxification of all fat-stored toxins and heavy metals; aid cardiovascular conditions, weight loss, and pain relief; and stimulate the immune system. Their Thermal Life Far Infrared Sauna is available in two- to four-person models.

Nutrition Education

Clayton College of Natural Health

2140 11th Ave. S, Suite 305
Birmingham, AL 35205
800–659–2426; 205–323–8246
communications@ccnh.edu; www.ccnh.edu

Clayton College offers degree programs in natural health and holistic nutrition through distance education. These programs are designed to provide students with a wide variety of tools with which they can educate others in achieving and maintaining health through the use of natural elements, such as proper diet, pure water, clean air, exercise, and rest. In addition to degree programs, CCNH offers certificate and/or concentration programs in herbal studies, nutrition and lifestyles, and iridology.

American College of Nutrition

300 S. Duncan Ave., Suite 225
Clearwater, FL 33755
Voice: 727–446–6086 / 7958; fax: 727–446–6202
office@am-coll-nutr.org

The American College of Nutrition was established in 1959 to promote scientific endeavor in the field of nutritional sciences.

RECOMMENDED BOOKS, MAGAZINES, NEWSLETTERS, AND WEB SITES

Here is a listing and a brief description of books, magazines, newsletters, and Web sites that are excellent companions for your Fast Track journey.

Books

The Fat Flush Plan
Ann Louise Gittleman, M.S., C.N.S.
McGraw-Hill, 2002

The Fat Flush Plan provides a three-phase program that can be used in conjunction with the Fast Track. Describing a more stringent and regimented program, this book is ideal for individuals who need everything laid out on a daily basis in terms of timing as well as menus for breakfast, lunch, dinner, and snacks.

The Fat Flush Cookbook
Ann Louise Gittleman, M.S., C.N.S.
McGraw-Hill, 2002

The cookbook provides over 200 recipes for breakfasts, snacks, lunches, dinners, desserts, and beverages that are compatible with the Fast Track.

The Fat Flush Fitness Plan
Ann Louise Gittleman, M.S., C.N.S., and Joanie Greggains
McGraw-Hill, 2003

Building on the workout component of the three-phase Fat Flush Plan, fitness expert Joanie Greggains designed specialty exercises that target the lymphatic system, which helps flush away fat. From rebounding, walking, and weight training to specially designed yoga stretches and deep breathing exercises.

How to Stay Young and Healthy in a Toxic World
Ann Louise Gittleman, M.S., C.N.S.
Keats Publishing, 1999

This book explores the four greatest hidden threats to health: sugar, parasites, heavy metals, and radiation. I teach you how to avoid these toxic invaders from your life and share the natural and even surprising solutions for myriad toxins that surround us in food and water and in our homes and workplaces.

It's All in Your Head—The Link between
Mercury Amalgams and Illness
Hal A. Huggins, D.D.S., M.S.
Avery, 1993

If mercury is one of the most poisonous substances known to man, why, then, do dentists routinely use it in amalgams to fill our teeth? That was the question asked by Hal Huggins over twenty years ago—and the same question is being asked today. Now, however, there is a growing chorus of dentists, researchers, and citizens adding their voices of concern. In this groundbreaking book, Huggins examines this question and more. What he finds may shock you, for in the face of overwhelming scientific evidence, the dangers of mercury exposure can no longer be ignored.

Uninformed Consent—The Hidden Dangers in Dental Care
Hal A. Huggins, D.D.S., M.S., and Thomas E. Levy, M.D., J.D.
Hampton Roads, 1999

Many "incurable" diseases may be incurable, but they may also be preventable. This prevention is accomplished not by using a multitude of modern miracle drugs, but directly by you. There is a price to pay. You must become informed and educated. You must be willing to discuss this situation because of the many legal implications and large sums of insurance money at risk.

Solving the MS Mystery: Help, Hope and Recovery
Hal A. Huggins, D.D.S., M.S.
Dragon Slayer, 2002

If, unfortunately, you have multiple sclerosis, or if you know someone who does, this definitive work in the field of autoimmune diseases is just what you have been looking for. Huggins had promised that, after treating 1,000 MS patients, he would write a book detailing the protocol that has worked to reverse autoimmune diseases. This is that book.

USA, Is There Poison in Your Mouth?
Hal A. Huggins, D.D.S., M.S.
Video: *60 Minutes*, 1989
www.drhuggins.com

This program got more inquiries than any other story *60 Minutes* has shown in over twenty years on the air, and *60 Minutes* got more threats from the ADA than they had received from anyone else during their history.

Hormone Deception
D. Lindsey Berkson
McGraw-Hill/Contemporary Books, 2002

This book reveals where hormone disruptors come from and how they affect adults, children, and the unborn child. It also gives you easy, practical tips for protecting your home and your family.

Going Against the Grain
Melissa Diane Smith
McGraw-Hill/Contemporary Books, 2002

Diets high in grains can lead to a host of health problems, such as obesity, diabetes, heart disease, fatigue, and more. This book outlines the disadvantages and potential dangers of eating various types of grains and provides practical, realistic advice on implementing a plan to cut back or eliminate grains on a daily basis.

Detoxify or Die
Sherry A. Rogers, M.D.
Prestige Publishing, 2002

It no longer matters what you call your disease. The label your doctor gives you is meaningless. What matters is what caused it. Learn how to find the underlying causes and get rid of them with the only proven ways to reverse the most hopeless diseases and slow down aging. You can reverse your disease and body damage.

Tired or Toxic?
Sherry A. Rogers, M.D.
Prestige Publishing, 1990

This is the first book that describes the mechanism, diagnosis, and treatment of chemical sensitivity, complete with scientific references. It is written for the layman and physician alike and explains the many vitamin, mineral, essential fatty acid, and amino acid analyses that help people detoxify everyday chemicals more efficiently and hence get rid of baffling symptoms.

Taste Life: The Organic Choice
David Richard
Vital Health Publishing, 1998

This book is written for current and potential consumers of organic foods. The perspectives of eighteen leaders, present and past, within the organic food movement serve to educate and inspire readers to upgrade their eating habits and enhance their health while they contribute to the environment and the sustainability of our food supply.

Our Children's Health
Bonnie C. Minsky and Lisa E. Holk
Vital Health Publishing, 2001

America is in the throes of a nutritional crisis—and children are at its very heart. Here is a book that forthrightly examines this problem and presents a positive, balanced approach to health and nutrition, offering hope to millions of undernourished, overmedicated children and their families.

GMO Free: Exposing the Hazards of Biotechnology to Ensure the Integrity of Our Food Supply
Vital Health Publishing, 2004

Clear, shocking, and compelling evidence for the worldwide banning of genetically modified foods. It is a profound indictment of our rush to commercialize genetic material.

Why Stomach Acid Is Good for You
Jonathan V. Wright, M.D., and Lane Lenard
M. Evans & Company, 2001

The authors use a combination of existing medical literature, clinical experience, and common sense to make the point that a stomach that is not functioning properly is associated not just with stomach problems but with many other medical problems as well (e.g., depression, autoimmune diseases, and asthma).

Politically Incorrect Nutrition
Michael Barbee
Vital Health Publishing, 2004

Using the most recent and objective scientific and clinical research data, this book reveals that much current nutritional dogma is based on outdated information or has been fabricated to satisfy vested corporate financial interests rather than to promote human health. Learn about these issues and more.

Magazines

Totalhealth for Longevity
165 N. 100 E, Suite #2
St. George, UT 84770–9963
800–788–7806
www.totalhealthmagazine.com

I am fortunate to serve as an associate editor for this magazine. It is a comprehensive voice in antiaging, longevity, and self-managed natural health. Lyle Hurd, publisher extraordinaire, strives to bring readers fresh new information and perspectives on all phases of longevity medicine so that you can make an educated decision on the quality of your life today . . . and tomorrow.

Taste for Life
86 Elm St.
Peterborough, NH 03458
603–924–9692
www.tasteforlife.com

This is one of the fastest growing in-store magazines for health food stores, natural product chains, food co-ops, and supermarkets nationwide. Its excellent articles on pertinent health issues offer readers an informative educational source on a variety of levels, including physical fitness. I sit on *Taste for Life*'s editorial board.

Let's Live
320 N. Larchmont Blvd.
P.O. Box 74908
Los Angeles, CA 90004
323–469–3901
www.letsliveonline.com

Boasting the largest circulation of all magazines in the natural foods industry, this is a monthly publication with cutting-edge articles about all facets of health and fitness.

First for Women
270 Sylvan Ave.
Englewood Cliffs, NJ 07632
800–938–8312
www.firstforwomen.com

This magazine speaks directly to women about their real-life needs, concerns, and interests. You can also read my monthly advice column, "Nutrition Know How."

Newsletters

The Sinatra Health Report
Published by Phillips Health, LLC
7811 Montrose Rd.
Potomac, MD 20854
800–211–7643
www.drsinatra.com

Stephen Sinatra, M.D., F.A.C.N., C.N.S., is a board-certified cardiologist and certified bioenergetic analyst with more than twenty years of experience in helping patients prevent and reverse heart disease. This newsletter is published monthly by Phillips Health. Sinatra, to his credit, is a big proponent of detoxification and many of his newsletters discuss current research in the environmental medicine arena.

The Woman's Health Letter
P.O. Box 467939
Atlanta, GA 31146–7939
800–728–2288

Nan Kathryn Fuchs, Ph.D., is the editor and my kind of nutritionist. Her comments regarding health, nutrition, and medicine as they relate to women are right on target.

Nutrition News
4108 Watkins Dr.
Riverside, CA 92507
909–784–7500; 800–784–7550
www.nutritionnews.com

Siri Khalsa is a wonderful veteran journalist who has been in the business of providing health education for over twenty-five years. Her easy-to-read newsletter covers a wide variety of contemporary and current topics. It is distributed in health food stores throughout the country, but you can subscribe directly.

Dr. Jonathan V. Wright's
Nutrition & Healing
Agora South, LLC
819 N. Charles St.
Baltimore, MD 21201
410–223–2611

This newsletter is dedicated to helping you keep yourself and your family healthy by the safest and most effective means possible. Every month, you'll get information about diet, vitamins, minerals, herbs, natural hormones, natural energies, and other substances and techniques to prevent and heal illness while prolonging your healthy life span.

ASSORTED WEB SITES

Liver

The following sites underscore the importance of the liver.

The American Liver Foundation
800–465–4837
www.liverfoundation.org

National Institute of Diabetes and
Digestive and Kidney Diseases
www.niddk.nih.gov

Celiac Disease

The following resources are available for those who want to learn more about gluten intolerance, gluten sensitivity, and full-blown celiac disease.

Celiac Disease and Gluten-Free Diet Support Center
www.celiac.com

This center provides important resources and information for people on gluten-free diets due to celiac disease, gluten intolerance, dermatitis herpetiformis, wheat allergy, or other health reasons.

The Celiac Disease Foundation
www.celiac.org

CDF provides support, information, and assistance to people affected by celiac disease/dermatitis herpetiformis (CD/DH). CDF works closely with health-care professionals and the pharmaceutical and medical industries. This cooperative effort puts CDF at the forefront of CD/DH care and research, helping aid and benefit those affected.

Celiac Sprue Association
877–272–4272
www.csaceliacs.org

CSA is a member-based, 501(c)(3) nonprofit support organization dedicated to helping individuals with celiac disease and dermatitis herpetiformis and their families worldwide through information, education, and research.

Environment

The following resources will keep you informed about the latest environmental issues and how they impact food choices.

Environmental Working Group
Washington, DC: 202–667–6982; Oakland, CA:
510–444–0973
www.ewg.org

The Fish List
info@seafoodchoices.com; www.thefishlist.org

The Seafood Choices Alliance
866–732–6673
www.seafoodchoices.com

Monterey Bay Aquarium Seafood Watch
24-hour information line: 831–648–4888; main number:
831–648–4800
www.mbayaq.org/cr/seafoodwatch.asp

FoodFirst—Institute for Food and Development Policy
510–654–4400
www.foodfirst.org

FoodIntegrity.com
www.foodintegrity.com

GOVERNMENT AGENCIES

National Organic Program
202–720–3252
www.ams.usda.gov/nop
This is the USDA Web site in which you will find the official definition of *organic* contained in volumes of pages. Basically, what you

need to know is that organic food is raised without synthetic pesticides, petroleum or sewage-sludge-based fertilizers, bioengineering, or ionizing radiation. Meat, poultry, eggs, and dairy products that are labeled organic must be derived from animals that are fed 100 percent organic feed without antibiotics or any growth hormones. A USDA inspector ensures that the farm where the food is produced meets quality standards before a product is labeled organic.

Generation Green
800–652–0827
www.generationgreen.org
This Web site keeps you informed about the latest government policies that affect food and the environment. Their quarterly newsletter keeps you up to date on the latest regulations and decisions regarding the food supply.

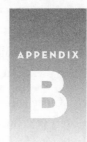

Visualizations for Your Fasting Day

Visualization: The Preparation

1. Find somewhere quiet and private, where you can enjoy at least fifteen minutes without interruption. No radio, TV, or phone—just you and your thoughts.

2. Sit in a comfortable position, with your back supported and your feet flat on the floor. Don't lie down, you might fall asleep! Let your hands rest loosely on your knees or in your lap without clasping or folding your hands and without crossing your feet.

3. Close your eyes and begin to breathe. Try to breathe in on a count of eight and out on the same count—or else work up from a two-count breath cycle to four, to six, and then to eight.

4. Breathe into your abdomen, letting one hand rest on your stomach to see how an inhale causes that area to expand while

an exhale allows it to collapse. Let your breath float in and out without forcing it.

Once you're breathing comfortably, you can begin your visualization. I've created two visualizations for you to experiment with. Each is designed to help you get in touch with a specific aspect of your relationship to food, eating, and hunger. Choose the one that instinctively seems right to you—or experiment with both over the course of your fasting day. I would suggest, however, that you allow at least two hours to go by between visualizations. Otherwise, you may begin to feel a bit on overload. Sample these visualizations, savor them, and don't gobble them down. That way, you'll get the most from each one.

I recommend making a tape of the visualization you've chosen, speaking slowly and pausing between each image, where I've put a series of dots. You can also consult the printed page—but you'll get much more out of the exercise if you continue breathing deeply, eyes closed, until you have finished.

When you've completed a visualization, I suggest you get out your journal and write about the experience. Visualizing is a powerful experience, and you need time to debrief, to process what you've learned, and to come to terms with how you feel. I've included a journal page for you to use after visualizing. Or just write whatever comes to mind.

Visualization: The Journey

OPTION 1: FAMINE AND FEAST

You are walking through the woods on a long journey. You've been walking quite a while, and you're pretty hungry. Feel the sensation of hunger in your stomach and experience it throughout your body . . . What happens to you when you get hungry? How do you feel? . . . What happens to your stomach, your muscles, your brain? . . . What happens elsewhere in your body? Pinpoint exactly where in your body you feel hungry, and how you feel when that sensation arises. . . .

Continue to see yourself walking through the woods, and continue to feel your hunger. What emotions go with your hunger? . . . Do you feel anxious? Angry? Frustrated? Sad? Excited? Strong? . . . What thoughts accompany your hunger? . . . What memories go with your hunger? . . .

As you continue through the woods, you come to a small clearing. A few feet away, resting on a table in the bright sunlight, is a huge feast. It has every kind of food, drink, and treat you could possibly want. What do you see on that table? . . . How do you feel when you see the food? . . . What do you think when you see the food? . . . Do any memories come to mind as you view this table full of delicious treats? What do you remember? . . .

See yourself moving toward the table. What do you do next? . . . How do you feel when you have reached the table? . . . What are you thinking about as you reach the table? . . .

See yourself eating and drinking whatever you want. Everything you want to eat or drink is on that table. As much as you want is on that table. Help yourself. See yourself eating and drinking, and notice how you feel. . . .

When you have eaten and drunk as much as you want, take a moment to see yourself again. What are you doing? . . . How are you feeling? . . . What do you want now? . . .

You realize that whoever supplied this magical table is ready to grant you one more wish. What do you wish for? . . . How do you feel about that wish? . . .

Take a moment to send a silent thank-you to whoever prepared that magical table for you . . . Send yourself a silent message as well . . . Then, when you are ready, walk through the woods until you have found your way home. When you are home, open your eyes.

OPTION 2: WHAT AM I HUNGRY FOR?

You are taking a long journey. At the moment, you have no particular goal or destination. You are simply walking through a place you enjoy, noticing the sights and sounds. Where are you? In the woods? By the beach? In a favorite city? On the street of a childhood neighborhood? In a strange place? A familiar one? . . . Allow yourself to visualize the place you would choose to pass a pleasant hour, simply walking and observing the world around you . . .

As you walk along, let your senses become sharper. What do you see? What colors, shapes, objects do you notice? Look at something you find beautiful and take a moment to savor what you see . . . What do you hear? What sounds reach your ears? Sounds of nature? Music? City traffic? People talking? Allow the sounds you enjoy most to float into your waiting ears . . . Continue walking as you notice your physical condition. Is the sun shining pleasantly? Is the ocean spray blowing over you in a fine mist? Are you wearing a warm coat in the brisk winter air? Allow yourself to experience your physical state . . . Then notice what you smell. Wood smoke? Salt water? Flowers? Freshly mowed grass? Allow yourself to enjoy the smells that reach your nose and mouth . . .

After you have fully enjoyed your walk, begin to allow yourself to wish for something more. You continue to walk, but now you begin to experience a new hunger. What is it for? Are you wishing for a companion by your side? A particular person or someone you imagine? . . . Or are you wishing for a destination to reach, a home, an exciting new workplace, a foreign country that you have never seen? . . . Perhaps you're longing for some condition in your life to change, wishing for more money or security, more recognition, more love? . . . Let the hungers come to the surface, one by one, and allow yourself to experience each one fully . . .

Say to yourself, "I want———" and finish the sentence in your mind. Now say it again: "I want———" . . . "I want———" . . . "I want———" . . . Continue to say "I want———" until you have named every wish that comes to the surface.

Continue walking in your ideal place. Allow your awareness to return to the sights, sounds, smells, and sensations you noticed before. As you feel your hunger for all the things you *don't* have, allow yourself to feel your satisfaction in the place you are as well. What is it like to feel both hungry and satisfied? . . . How do you feel? . . . What are you thinking? . . . What memories come to mind? . . .

Give yourself a moment to say a grateful good-bye to the beautiful place you have just visited. Take one last look at the things you love to see . . . Listen one last time to the things you love to hear . . . Feel your physical presence and enjoy what you feel . . . Smell the odors and scents that reach your nose and mouth and allow yourself to enjoy them, too . . . Remind yourself that you can return to this place anytime you want to, simply by shutting your eyes.

Allow yourself the time to make any promises you wish to yourself . . . Then see yourself walking home. When you have found your way home, open your eyes.

YOUR FAST TRACKER JOURNAL:
AFTER VISUALIZING

Now that I've completed my visualization, I realize that

_____

_____

_____

_____

Right now, I'm feeling

_____

_____

_____

_____

Something I didn't expect to learn from visualizing was

_____

_____

_____

I will make use of what I learned today by

_____

_____

_____

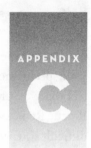

Bach Flower
Remedies

The Bach Flower Remedies were developed in the 1930s by British bacteriologist Dr. Edward Bach to help people relieve troubling mental states such as loneliness, uncertainty, and fear. Grateful residents of England, Europe, and the United States have been using them ever since. Today, the Bach Flower Remedies are available online, in fine health food stores, and even in some drugstores. While there are other botanicals that may seem similar, the Bach Flower Remedies are the ones I have found to be the most effective.

On nonfast days, I recommend taking them in a half-filled glass of water or placing three or four drops under the tongue. If you want to remove the minute traces of alcohol used to extract the essence of these herbs and flowers, let a few drops sit for a few minutes in warm (not hot) water and then drink. If you choose to use them during your One-Day Detox Diet, you might have a slight reaction to the alcohol, so just dab a few drops on your wrist.

I recommend choosing a maximum of four remedies based on your specific needs and using them as frequently as needed until you feel that you are centered and at peace. My own personal favorite is Rescue Remedy, which has gotten me and my clients through many a difficult situation, from the sudden death of a loved one to a sleepless night. You can experiment to find which formula is your personal choice, but here are a few that I have come to rely on.

- **Bach's Rescue Remedy:** This remedy helps you move through numbness, trauma, panic, terror, tension, and other acute states. It's very calming for everything from everyday frustration to major tragedy.

- **Beech:** This is the formula to use when you're feeling critical, intolerant, even arrogant. It will help soften the rough edges and let you get in touch with a more tolerant and generous side of your nature.

- **Centaury:** If you've ever felt like you say yes too easily and no too rarely, this is the formula for you. It's designed to help repair weakness of will and to support your efforts to stop being exploited or imposed on.

- **Elm:** During the times when you feel temporarily overcome by inadequacy, this formula can help you regain your normal sense of competence. It will support your feelings of being capable and effective.

- **Holly:** Have you ever found yourself feeling jealous, vengeful, or envious? Do your suspicions sometimes get the better of you? Can you occasionally behave in a way that is downright hateful? Then holly is the remedy for you, to help you connect to your more loving and trusting side.

- **Impatiens:** The name says it all: when you're behaving in an impatient, irritable way, a few drops of this remedy will calm you right down.[1]

Notes

CHAPTER 1

1. Haas, Elson, *The Detox Diet* (Berkeley, CA: Celestial Arts, 2004), p. 108.
2. Khalsa, Siri, "Pollution Protection," *Nutrition News* 23, no. 7 (2003).
3. Guthrie, Catherine, "Can You Lighten Your Toxic Load?" *Alternative Medicine* (June 2003), p. 72.
4. Ibid., p. 75.
5. Health Sciences Institute, *Rebuild, Rejuvenate & Reform Your Health* (Baltimore: Institute of Health Sciences, 2003), p. 10; citing Macintosh, A., and Ball, K., "The Effects of a Short Program of Detoxification in Disease-free Individuals," *Alternative Therapies in Health and Medicine* 6, no. 4 (2000), pp. 70–76.
6. Ibid., citing Bland, J. S., Barrager, E., Reedy, R. G., and Bland, K., "A Medical Food-Supplemented Detoxification Program in the Management of Chronic Health Problems," *Alternative Therapies in Health and Medicine* 1, no. 5 (1995), pp. 62–71.
7. Ibid., citing Liska, D. J., "The Detoxification Enzyme System," *Alternative Medicine Review* 3, no. 3 (1998), pp. 187–98.
8. Guthrie, "Can You Lighten Your Toxic Load?," p. 72.
9. Adapted from Haas, *The Detox Diet,* p. 113.

CHAPTER 2

1. I am indebted to Haas, Elson M., *The Detox Diet* (Berkeley, CA: Celestial Arts, 2004), pp. 24–25, and to Lipman, Frank, and

Gunning, Stephanie, *Total Renewal* (New York: Jeremy Tarcher, 2003), pp. 208–9, for some of the information on which these quizzes in this book are based. You can find more details on toxicity and particular organs in my own *The Living Beauty Detox Program* (San Francisco: HarperCollins San Francisco, 2000), pp. 40–47.

2. Health Sciences Institute, *Rebuild, Rejuvenate & Reform Your Health* (Baltimore: Institute of Health Sciences, 2003), p. 4.

3. Sinatra, Stephen, *The Sinatra Health Report,* March 2003, pp. 1–2.

4. Khalsa, Siri, "Pollution Protection," *Nutrition News* 23, no. 7 (2003).

5. Berkson, D. Lindsey, *Hormone Deception: How Everyday Foods and Products Are Disrupting Your Hormones—And How to Protect Yourself and Your Family* (New York: McGraw-Hill, 2001), p. 233.

6. Baillie-Hamilton, Paula, *The Body Restoration Plan* (New York: Avery, 2002, 2003), p. 29; citing Stellman, S. D., et al., "Adipose and Serum Levels of Organochlorinated Pesticides and PCB Residues in Long Island Women: Association with Age and Body Mass," *American Journal of Epidemiology* [Abstract] (1997), p. 81; Ashby, J., et al., "Lack of Effects for Low-Dose Levels of Bisphenoal A and Diethylstilbestrol on the Prostate Gland of CF1 Mice Exposed in Utero," *Regulatory Toxicology and Pharmacology* 30, no. 2, pt. 1 (1999), pp. 156–66; Hardin, B. D., et al., "Evaluation of 60 Chemicals in a Preliminary Developmental Toxicity Test," *Carcinogens, Mutagens and Teratogens* 7 (1987), pp. 29–48; and Clark, D. R., "Bats and Environmental Contaminants: A Review" [U.S. Department of the Interior: Fish and Wildlife Service, Special Scientific Report], *Wildlife* 235 (1981), pp. 1–29.

7. Ibid., pp. 26–27; citing Heeremans, A., et al., "Elimination Profile of Methylthiouracil in Cows after Oral Administration," *Analyst* 123 (1988), pp. 2625–28; Sawaya, A. L., and Lunn, P. G., "Lowering of Plasma Triiodothyronine Level and Sympathetic Activity Does Not Alter Hypoalbuminaemiain Rats Fed a Low Protein Diet," *British Journal of Nutrition* 79, no. 5 (1998), pp. 455–62.

8. Ibid., pp. 31–32; citing Antonio, M. T., et al., "Neurochemical Changes in Newborn Rat's Brain after Gestational Cadmium and Lead Exposure," *Toxicology Letters* 104, nos. 1–2 (1999), pp. 1–9; Field, E. A., et al., "Developmental Toxicology Evaluation of Diethyl

and Dimethyl Phthalate in Rats," *Teratology* 48, no. 1 (1993), pp. 33–44; Gupta, B. N., et al., "Effects of a Polybrominated Biphenyl Mixture in the Rat and Mouse: I. Six-Month Exposure," *Toxicology and Applied Pharmacology* 68, no. 1 (1983), pp. 1–18.

9. Health Sciences Institute, *Rebuild, Rejuvenate & Reform Your Health*, p. 6; citing Baillie-Hamilton, P. F., "Chemical Toxins: A Hypothesis to Explain the Global Obesity Epidemic," *Journal of Alternative and Complementary Medicine* 8, no. 2 (2002), pp. 185–192.

10. Ibid.; citing Deichmann, W. B., MacDonald, W. E., and Cubit, D. A., "Dieldrin and DDT in the Tissues of Mice Fed Aldrin and DDT for Seven Generations," *Archives of Toxicology* 34, no. 3 (1975), pp. 173–82.

11. Ibid.; citing Villeneuve, D. C., van Logten, M. J., Den Tonkelaar, E. M., Greve, P. A., Vos, J. G., et al., "Effect of Food Deprivation on Low Level Hexachlorobenzene Exposure in Rats," *Science of the Total Environment* 8, no. 2 (1977), pp. 186–97.

12. Baillie-Hamilton, *The Body Restoration Plan*, pp. 41–42, 45, 46; citing Chadwick, R. W., et al., "Effects of Age and Obesity on the Metabolism of Lindane by Black a/a, Yellow Avy/a, and Pseudoagouti Avy/a Phenotypes of (ys xvy) FI Hybrid Mice," *Journal of Toxicoloty and Environmental Health* 16 (1985), pp. 771–96; Guengerich, F. P., "Influence of Nutrients and Other Dietary Materials on Cytochrome P-450 Enzymes," *American Journal of Clinical Nutrition* 61, no. 3 (1995), pp. 651s–58s; Schildkraut, J. M., et al., "Environmental Contaminants and Body Fat Distribution," *Cancer Epidemiology, Biomarkers & Prevention* 8 (1999), pp. 179–83.

13. Lee, John, Hanley, Jesse, and Hopkins, Virginia, *What Your Doctor May Not Tell You about Premenopause* (New York: Warner, 1999), pp. 44–47. See also my own *Why Am I Always So Tired?* (San Francisco: Harper San Francisco, 2000).

14. Lee et al., *What Your Doctor May Not Tell You about Premenopause*, p. 48.

15. Ibid.

16. Ibid.

17. Berkson, *Hormone Deception*, pp. 220, 222.

18. Ibid., p. 218.

19. Ibid., p. 224.

20. Health Sciences Institute, *Rebuild, Rejuvenate & Reform Your Health,* p. 6; citing Olea, N., Pazos, P., and Esposito, J. "Inadvertent Exposure to Xenoestrogens," *European Journal of Cancer Prevention* 7, Supplement 1 (1998), S17–S23.

CHAPTER 3

1. Barbee, Michael, *Politically Incorrect Nutrition* (Ridgefield, CT: Connecticut: Vital Health Publishing, 2004), p. 86.

2. Berkson, D. Lindsey, *Hormone Deception: How Everyday Foods and Products Are Disrupting Your Hormones—And How to Protect Yourself and Your Family* (New York: McGraw-Hill, 2001), p. 218.

3. Baillie-Hamilton, Paula, *The Body Restoration Plan* (New York: Avery, 2002, 2003), p. 151.

4. Ibid.; citing Guengerich, F. P., "Influence of Nutrients and Other Dietary Materials on Cytochrome P-450 Enzymes," *American Journal of Clinical Nutrition* 61, no. 3 (1995), 651s–658s.

5. Wright, Jonathan, and Lenard, Jane, *Why Stomach Acid Is Good for You* (New York: M. Evans & Co., 2001), p. 130.

6. Smith, Melissa Diane, *Going against the Grain: How Reducing and Avoiding Grains Can Revitalize Your Health* (New York: Contemporary Books, 2002), pp. 68–69; citing Gerarduzzi, T., et al., "Celiac Disease in U.S.A. among Risk Groups and the General Population in U.S.A." [Abstract], *Journal of Pediatric Gastroenterology and Nutrition* 31, Supplement (2000): S29.

7. Ibid., pp. 69–70.

8. Ibid., pp. 80–83; citing Nellen, H., et al., "Treatment of Human Immunodeficiency Virus Enteropathy with a Gluten-Free Diet," *Archives of Internal Medicine* 160 (2000), p. 244; Michaelsson, G., et al., "Psoriasis Patients with Antibodies to Gliadin Can Be Improved by a Gluten-Free Diet," *British Journal of Dermatology* 142 (2000), pp. 44–51; Hadjivassiliou, M., Gibson, A., and Davies-Jones, G. A. B., "Does Cryptical Gluten Sensitivity Play a Part in Neurological Illness?," *Lancet* 347 (1996), pp. 369–71; Collin, P., et al., "Celiac Disease, Brain Atrophy, and Dementia," *Neurology* 41 (1991), pp.

372–75; Hadjivassiliou, M., et al., "Headaches and CNS White Matter Abnormalities with Gluten Sensitivity," *Neurology* 56 (2001), pp. 385–88; Gobbi, G., et al., "Coeliac Disease, Epilepsy, and Cerebral Calcifications," *Lancet* 340 (1992), pp. 439–43; Ventura, A., et al., "Coeliac Disease, Folic Acid Deficiency and Epilepsy with Cerebral Calcifications," *Acta Paediatrica Scandinavica* 80 (1991), pp. 559–62; Luostarinen, L., Pirttila, T., and Collin, P., "Coeliac Disease Presenting with Neurological Disorders," *European Neurology* 42 (1999), pp. 132–35; Reichelt, K. L., and Landmark, J., "Specific Antibody Increases in Schizophrenia," *Biological Psychiatry* 37 (1995), pp. 410–13; and Cade, R., et al., "Autism and Schizophrenia: Intestinal Disorders," *Nutritional Neuroscience* 3 (2000), pp. 57–72.

9. Eades, Michael, and Dan, Mary, "Snack-Food Nation," *LowCarb Living* (March/April 2004), p. 52.

10. Davidson, T. L., and Swithers, S. E., "A Pavlovian Approach to the Study of Obesity," *International Journal of Obesity* 28, no. 7 (2004), pp. 933–35.

CHAPTER 4

1. Colbert, Don, *Toxic Relief* (Lake Mary, FL: Siloam, 2001, 2003), pp. 134–35.

2. Adapted from Health Sciences Institute, *Rebuild, Rejuvenate & Reform Your Health* (Baltimore: Institute of Health Sciences, 2003), p. 16.

CHAPTER 5

1. Barbee, Michael, *Politically Incorrect Nutrition* (Ridgefield, CT: Vital Health Publishing, 2004), pp. 1–6.

CHAPTER 6

1. Bomser, J., Madhavi, D. L., Singletary, K., and Smith, M. A., "Anti-Cancer Activity of Cranberry Extracts," *Planta Medica* 62 (1996), pp. 212–16; Kandil, F. E., Smith, M. A., Robers, R. B., Pepin, M., Song, L. L., Pezzuto, J. M., and Seigler, D. S., "Composition of a

Chemopreventive Ornithin Decarboxylase (ODC) Activity," *Journal of Agricultural and Food Chemistry* 50, no. 5 (2002), pp. 1063–69; Narayanan, B. A., Narayanan, N. K., Stoner, G. D., and Bullock, B. P., "Interactive Gene Expression Pattern in Prostate Cancer Cells Exposed to Phenolic Antioxidant Ellagic Acid," *Anticancer Research* 21 (2001), pp. 359–64; Narayanan, B. A., Geoffrey, O., Willingham, C. M., Re, G. G., and Nixon, D. W., "(WAFLCIPI) Expression and Its Possible Role in GI Arrest and Apoptosis," *Cancer Letters* 136 (1999), pp. 215–21; Festa, T., Aglitti, T., Duranti, G., Ricordy, R., Perticone, P., and Cozzi, R., "Strong Antioxidant Activity of Ellagic Acid in Mammalian Cells In Vitro Revealed by the Comet Assay," *Anticancer Research* 21, no. 6A (2001), pp. 3903–8; Bilyk, A., and Sapers, G. A., "Varietal Differences in the Quercitin, Kaempferol, and Myricetin Contents of Highbush Blueberry, Cranberry, and Thornless Blackberry Fruits," *Journal of Agricultural and Food Chemistry* 34 (1986), pp. 585–88; Verma, A. K., et al., "Inhibition of 7,12-Dimethylben(a)anthracene- and N-Nitrosemethylurea-Induced Rat Mammary Cancer by Dietary Flavonol, Quercitin," *Cancer Research* 48, no. 20 (1988), pp. 5754–58; and Guthrie, N., "Effect of Cranberry Juice and Products on Human Breast Cancer Cell Growth," *Journal of the Federation of American Societies for Experimental Biology* 14, no. 4 (2000), p. A771.

2. Centers for Disease Control and Prevention, "Facts about Cardiovascular Disease," available at www.cdc.gov/oe/oc/media/fact/cardiova.htm, accessed September 3, 2002; Reed, J., "Cranberry Flavonoids, Atherosclerosis and Cardiovascular Health," *Critical Reviews in Food Science and Nutrition* 42, Supplement (2002), pp. 301–16; Princen, H. M. G., Feskens, E. J. M., Hollman, P. C. H., Katan, M. B., and Kromhout, D., "Dietary Antioxidant Flavonoids and Risk of Coronary Heart Disease: The Zuptphen Elderly Study," *Lancet* 342 (1993), pp. 1007–11; Ross, R., "Mechanisms of Disease: Atherosclerosis—An Inflammatory Disease," *New England Journal of Medicine* 340, no. 2 (1999), pp. 115–26; Fuster, V., Ross R., and Topol, E. J., eds., *Atherosclerosis and Coronary Artery Disease* (Philadelphia: Lippincott-Raven Publishers, 1996); Wang, P., Du, C., and Francis, F., "Isolation and Characterization of Polyphenolic

Compounds in Cranberries," *Journal of Food Science* 43 (1978), pp. 1402–4; Howell, A. B., Vorsa, N., Der Mardarosian, A., and Foo, L. Y., "Inhibition of the Adherence of P-Finbriated *Escherichia coli* to Uropithelial-Cell Surfaces by Proanthocyanidin Extracts from Cranberries," *New England Journal of Medicine* 339, no. 15 (1998), pp. 1085–86; Weiss, E. I., Lev-Dor, R., Sharon, N., and Oftek, I., "Inhibitory Effect of High-Molecular-Weight Constituent of Cranberry on Adhesion of Oral Bacateria," *Critical Reviews in Food Science and Nutrition* 42, Supplement (2002), pp. 285–92; and Youdim, K. A., McDonald, J., Kalt, W., and Joseph, J. A., "Potential Role of Dietary Flavonoids in Reducing Microvascular Endothelium Vulnerability to Oxidative and Inflammatory Insults," *Journal of Nutritional Biochemistry* 13, no. 5 (2002), pp. 282–88.

3. The Cranberry Institute, *Cranberry Health News* 2, no. 3 (n.d.), p. 4.

4. Reed, "Cranberry Flavonoids, Atherosclerosis and Cardiovascular Health"; and Reed, J. D., Porter, M. I., Krueger, C. G., and Wiebe, D. A., "Cranberry Proanthocyanidins Differ in the Inhibition of Cupric-Induced Oxidation of Human Low Density Lipoprotein," *Journal of the Federation of American Societies for Experimental Biology* 15 (2001), p. LB54.

5. Dorrell, N., Crabtree, J. E., and Wren, B. W., "Host-Bacterial Interactions and the Pathogenesis of *Helicobacter pylori* infection," *Trends in Microbiology* 6 (1998), pp. 379–81; and Blaser, M. J., "*Helicobacter pylori* Eradication and Its Implications for the Future," *Ailment Pharmacological Therapies* 11 (1997), pp. 103–7.

6. The Cranberry Institute, *Cranberry Health News* 2, no. 2 (winter 2004), p. 1.

7. Reid, B., "The Role of Cranberry and Probiotics in Intestinal and Urogenital Tract Health," *Critical Reviews of Food Science and Nutrition* 42, Supplement (2002), pp. 293–300; Howell, A., and Foxman, B., "Cranberry Juice and Adhesion of Antibiotic-Resistant Bacteria," *Journal of American Medical Association* 287, no. 23 (2002), pp. 3082–83.

8. Moore, W. E., and Moore, L. V., "The Bacteria of Periodontal Disease," *Periodontology 20001* 5 (1994), pp. 66–77; and Weiss, et al., "Inhibitory Effect of High-Molecular-Weight Constituent of Cranberry on Adhesion of Oral Bacteria."

9. Vinson, J. A., Su, X., Zuik, L., and Bose, P., "Phenol Antioxidant Quantity and Quality in Foods: Fruits," *Journal of Agricultural and Food Chemistry* 49 (2001), pp. 5315–21; Vinson, J. A., Dabbagh, Y. A., Serry, M. M., and Jang, J., "Plant Flavonoids, Especially Tea Flavonols, Are Powerful Antioxidants Using an In Vitro Oxidation Model for Heart Disease," *Journal of Agricultural and Food Chemistry* 43 (1995), pp. 2800–2; and Vinson, J. A., Su, X., and Zuik, L., "Phenol Antioxidant Quantity and Quality in Foods: Vegetables," *Journal of Agricultural and Food Chemistry* 46 (1998), pp. 3630–34.

10. Jarvill-Taylor, Karalee J., Anderson, Richard A., and Graves, Donald J., "A Hydroxychalcone Derived from Cinnamon Functions as a Mimetic for Insulin in 3T3-L1 Adipocytes," *Journal of the American College of Nutrition* 20, no. 4 (2001), pp. 327–36.

11. Gittleman, Ann Louse, *Fat Flush Foods* (New York: McGraw-Hill, 2004), pp. 100–1; citing Colquhoun, E., "Pungent Principles of Ginger (*Zingiber officinale*) Are Thermogenic in the Perfused Rat Hindlimb," *The International Journal of Obesity* 16 (1992).

CHAPTER 7

1. Adapted from Lamothe, Denise, *The Taming of the Chew* (New York: Penguin, 1998), pp. 166–67.

CHAPTER 8

1. Colbert, Don, *Toxic Relief* (Lake Mary, FL: Siloam, 2001, 2003), pp. 140–43.

CHAPTER 9

1. Mars, Brigitte, *Rawsome!* (North Bergen, NJ: Basic Health Publications, 2004), p. 9.

2. Ibid., p. 10.

3. Williams, David G., "Longevity Is on the Menu," *Alternatives for the Health-Conscious Individual* 10, no. 12 (June 2004), pp. 89–90.

4. Joachim, David, and Davis, Rochelle, *Fresh Choices* (New York: Rodale/St. Martin's Press, 2004), p. 11.

5. Gittleman, Ann Louise, *The Fat Flush Foods* (New York: McGraw-Hill, 2004), pp. 125–26.

6. Joachim and Davis, *Fresh Choices,* p. 153.

7. Ibid., pp. 152–53, 156.

8. Ibid., pp. 151–52.

9. Ibid., p. 123.

10. Merrell, Kathy, "Hungry for Organic," *Real Simple* (September 2004), pp. 173–79.

11. Joachim and Davis, *Fresh Choices,* p. 97; citing Environmental Working Group, "PCBs in Farmed Salmon: Factory Methods, Unnatural Results," July 2003, available at www.ewg.org/reports/ farmed PCBs/es.php.

12. Ibid., pp. 101, 104.

13. Ibid., pp. 97–98.

14. Ibid., pp. 182–83.

15. Ibid., p. 65.

16. Ibid., pp. 35–37, 66.

17. Ibid., pp. 31–37, 59–68.

18. Huggins, Hal A., *Detoxification* (Colorado Springs, CO, self-published), pp. 16–18.

19. Gittleman, Ann Louise, *How to Stay Young and Healthy in a Toxic World* (Los Angeles: Keats, 1999), pp. 168–71.

20. Barbee, Michael, *Politically Incorrect Nutrition* (Ridgefield, CT: Vital Health Publishing, 2004), p. 91; citing Kopp, W. P., "Effects of Microwaves on Humans," *Journal of Natural Science* 1, no. 1 (1998), pp. 42–43.

APPENDIX C

1. Information taken from Gittleman, Ann Louise, *How to Stay Young and Healthy in a Toxic World* (Los Angeles: Keats, 1999), pp. 175–79.

Index